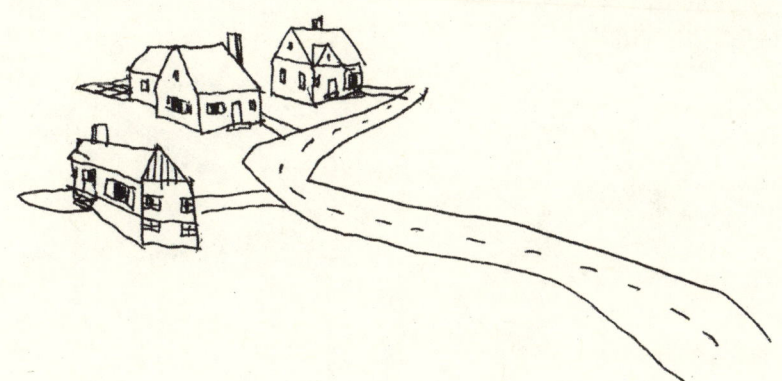

STROKELAND
A MEMOIR

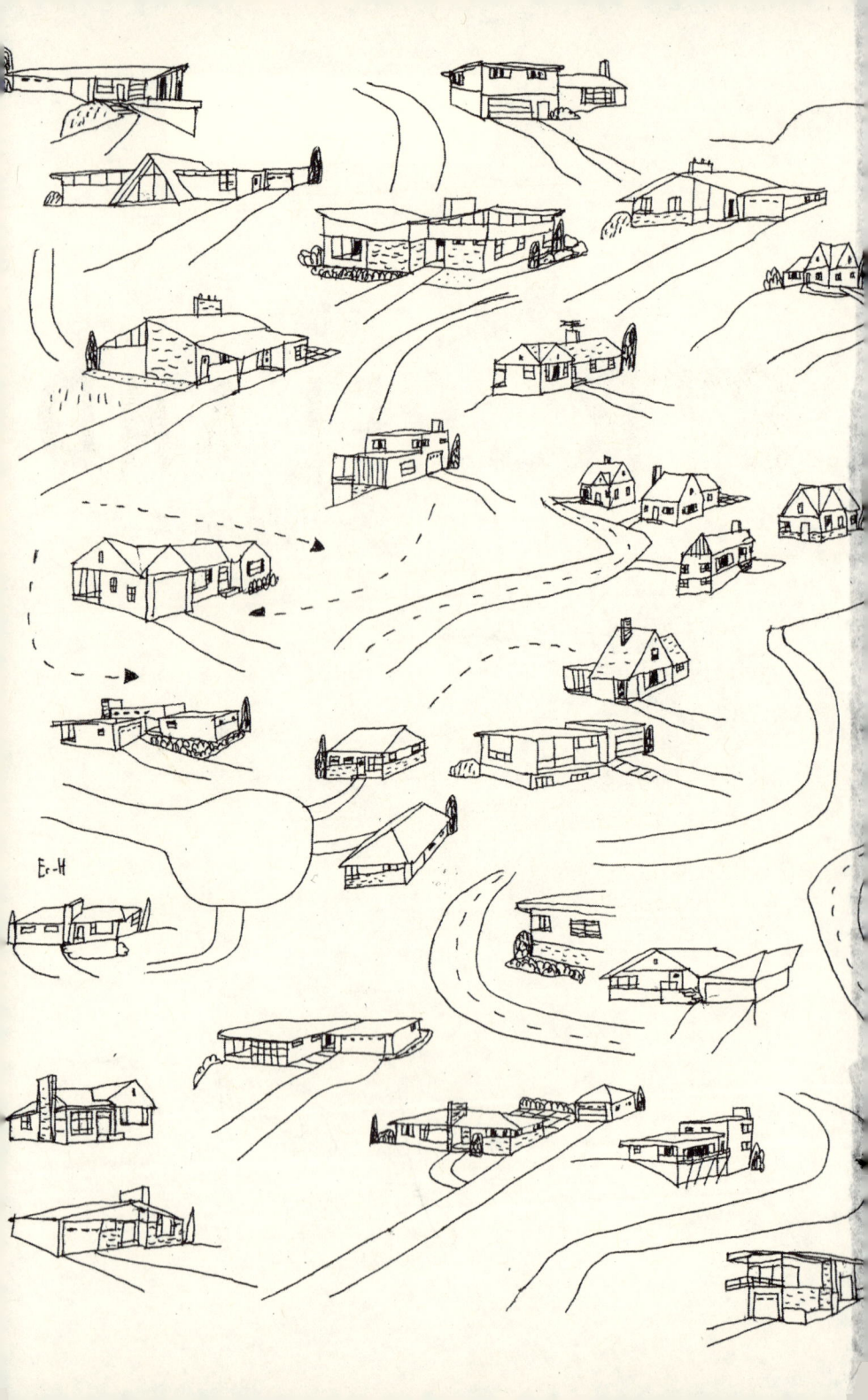

STROKELAND
A MEMOIR

MY HUSBAND'S MIDLIFE
BRAINSTORM
AND ITS AMBIVALENT
AFTERMATH

LYNETTE LAMB

© 2021 Lynette Lamb

ISBN 978-1-7366972-0-7

Cover illustration and design by Eric Hanson

Book design by Brian Donahue/bedesigninc.com

Author photo by Belen Fleming/Belu Photography

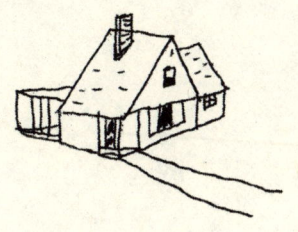

For Robert,
whose amazing work ethic
and abiding good humor
have never failed him

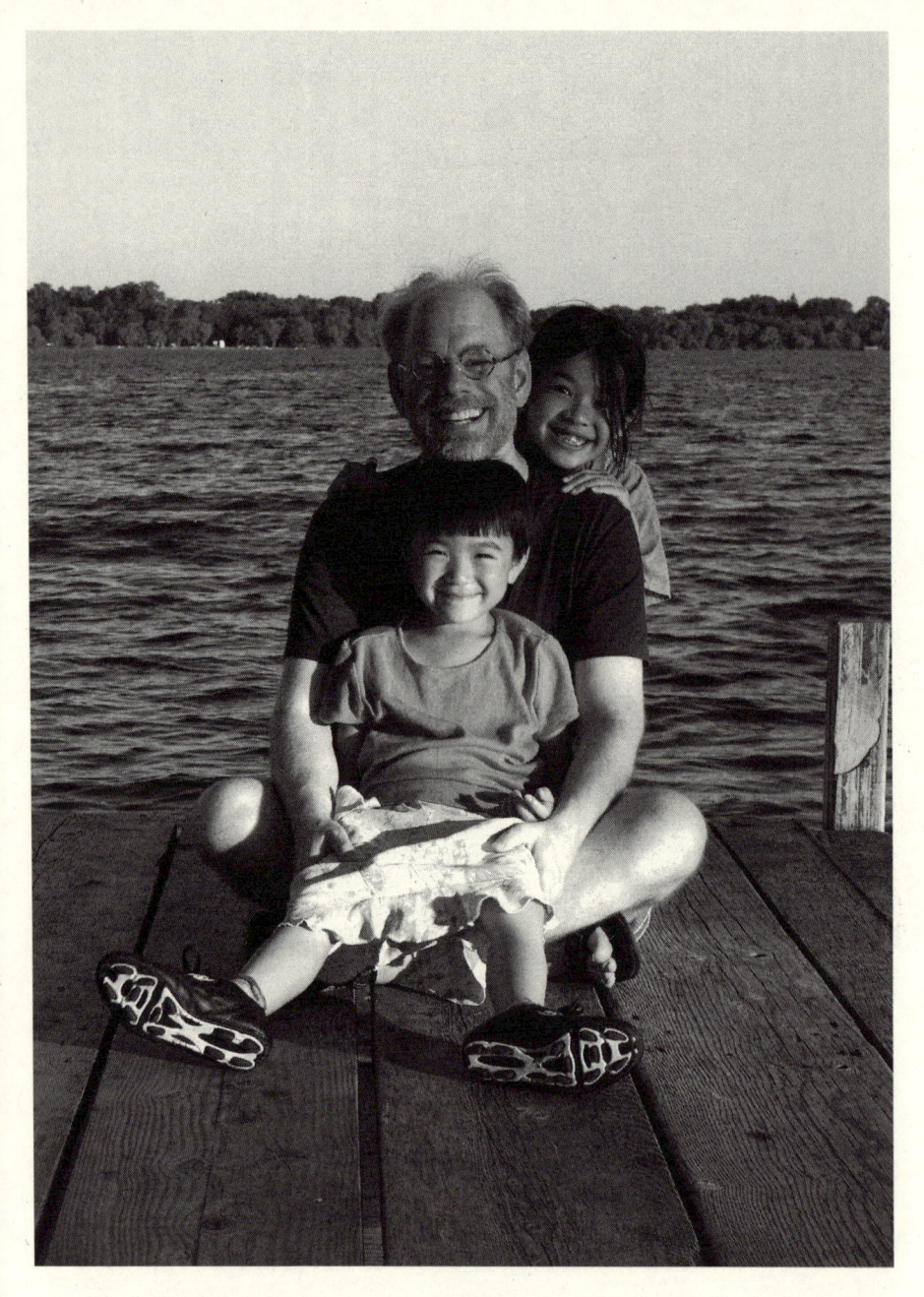

On a regular Lake Harriet visit in 2005 (from back: Grace, Rob, and Julia)
PHOTO BY LYNETTE LAMB

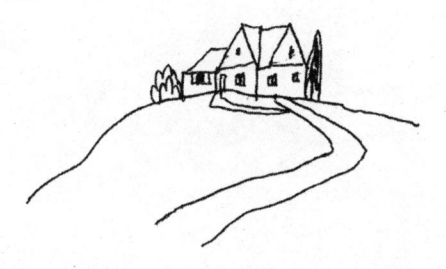

A HUNDRED YEARS AGO, having a stroke meant certain death. Over the intervening decades, decreasing stroke mortality has been one of our nation's major public health victories. In the first decade of this century, survival rates took yet another upward swing.

My husband, Robert Gerloff, survived a massive stroke in 2006; had he suffered the same blood clot to the brain even 10 years earlier, he probably would have died. Like other families in this situation, we are grateful for the medical care he received, which meant he returned to us instead.

However, Rob—like most stroke survivors—came home utterly altered. One of the largely unknown stories of this public health triumph is what a stroke survivor's life looks like after the medical emergency has passed, and what that personal transformation means for him and his family.

This memoir is about Robert, yes, but it is more about me as his caretaker, and how this catastrophic incident bifurcated our lives. In our family, we always talk about life before Rob's stroke and after, because nothing has been the same since. The following represents my attempt to tell that story, one that so often goes untold.

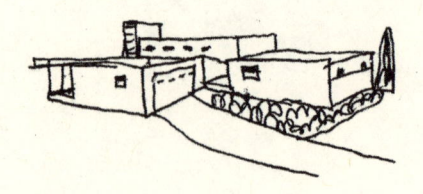

JULY 16, 2006

It's Sunday afternoon, and I've been out of town for the weekend. When I come up the driveway, Julia and Grace run down to meet my car. They're in grade school. They're laughing, saying, "Come see Dad. He's playing a game upstairs. He's being funny." I laugh along, climbing the stairs.

What I see in the bathroom isn't funny. Rob is lying on the floor in the fetal position, twitching, unconscious. I am incredulous to see my energetic, vital husband incapacitated. A sense of unreality washes over me. "Dad started to fall when we were fighting," Grace tells me. At 10, she is the older, more verbal sister. "We helped him lie down. We gave him a pillow. We tried your cell phone. We rode our bikes around the block. I had Julia watch a movie," said Grace. "Dad was talking funny."

I start to yell, "Get me a phone. Call 911. Where's the phone?" This is 2006, before our cell phones were permanently attached to us, and I cannot find our portable land line. I run downstairs and make a call I can no longer remember.

Soon the EMTs are charging upstairs, asking questions I cannot answer. The worst one is, "How long has he been lying there?" The girls don't know. I don't know. A late adapter to cell phones, I had mine turned off for the entire five-hour drive from Madison, Wisconsin, to Minneapolis. Make that six hours: Exhausted from a weekend spent with my parents, reeling from my mother's recent lung cancer diagnosis, I had stopped at a rest area to nap. When I called the home line from a gas station an hour away, no one answered.

I make a frantic call to our next-door neighbor, asking her to stay with the girls, and rush off to Fairview Southdale Hospital, following the ambulance. I am worried, naturally, but assume that Rob's collapse is related to his blood sugar levels, which have been hovering in dangerous pre-diabetes territory for months. I assume he has finally fallen, quite literally, into diabetes itself. Both Rob's father and his paternal grandmother Nielsen had diabetes, despite being small, thin people like Robert. It ran viciously and persistently in the Nielsen family. It was the only thing I could think of. What else could drop an otherwise healthy 45-year-old man? I tell myself that with a little insulin and some diet changes, he will be as good as new.

As far as I can piece together from the girls' rambling narratives, it has been several hours since he collapsed.

There was no blood, no broken bones, so they didn't think they should call 911. I couldn't think straight, but I did know this: I must always remind them that it wasn't their fault. If anyone was to blame, it was me. They took care of him the very best they could.

As for Rob, although he appeared to be unconscious, years later he told us that he was actually drifting in and out of consciousness, and that many thoughts flew through his head over those hours. The first thing he thought of, which made us laugh when he told us later, was, "Damn it, now we won't be able to remodel the kitchen!" After a dozen years of living with cheap plastic cabinets, a nasty vinyl floor, and other indignities, Rob—a residential architect—had just days earlier finished the drawings for a beautiful new room.

He also thought about money and was comforted by the memory of having purchased private disability insurance, which guaranteed our family a set monthly income until Rob reached 65. It was an expensive addition to an already tight budget, but a wise financial counselor had strongly urged him to buy it, pointing out that people in their forties and fifties were more likely to become disabled than to die.

Most painfully, Rob later told us that he instantly knew that whatever was happening to him was catastrophic and that he would never work again. And, of course, he wondered when the paramedics would arrive. Incapable of speech, he couldn't tell the girls to call for help, and they didn't know what to do. So they made him comfortable—putting a pillow under his head, placing a rubber duck in his hand when they saw his nails biting into his palm—and waited for me to return, a wait that was somewhere between two and four hours. It haunts me still to think of Rob lying on that bathroom floor, losing and regaining consciousness, thoughts and worries spinning through his already diminished mind.

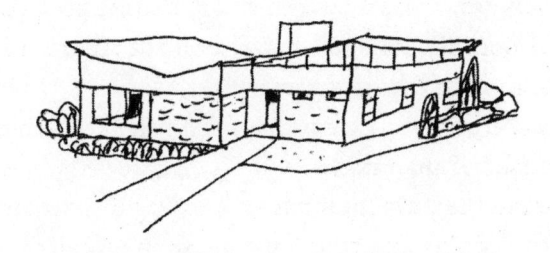

THE HOSPITAL

I had been in my ER alcove just half an hour when a doctor came to tell me that Rob had suffered an ischemic stroke, which is when a blood clot hits the brain. (Later I would learn to distinguish this from a hemorrhagic stroke, a brain bleed.) The doctor immediately began firing questions at me: How many hours had it been since he had the stroke? Was it two, three, four? When I couldn't answer, they decided it was too risky to use the clot-dissolving drug and should instead try a thrombectomy, which is when a surgeon snakes a tube up through the groin to the brain in an attempt to claw out the clot.

Since it was a Sunday afternoon in mid-summer, a neuro-interventionist had to be called in from whatever boat ride or picnic he was enjoying; that took more than an hour. Although they held out some hope that the claw might work, the neurologist cautioned me, "I must tell you, Mrs. Gerloff, your husband's condition is very serious."

What? A stroke? Rob was just 45 years old, had average blood pressure, wasn't overweight, sedentary, or a smoker—all of the qualities I associated with strokes. The only stroke survivor I even knew was a 70-year-old part-time minister at our church, a man whose slurred words made me think he was drunk the first time I heard him deliver a sermon. I knew nothing else about strokes, except that most people who have them are decades older than Rob.

And then there was that nagging question—how long? How long had it been? I would hear that question repeatedly over the next few weeks, and each time, excruciatingly, I would have no answer. The girls didn't know, and I certainly did not. Rob could have laid on that bathroom floor for one hour or six hours—or any length of time in between.

I had been out of reach while I drove home from Madison. Of course, when I finally got home and found Rob unconscious, I asked the girls how long it had been since their Dad had fallen, but they were grade-schoolers and thus largely unaware of time and its passing.

Why, oh why, was I such a techno-idiot? The girls told me they had repeatedly called my cell phone. Why had I turned it off? Why was I incapable of retrieving its messages? What if? What if? What if? resounded through my brain like a drumbeat for weeks afterward.

I was soon joined by an unidentified hospital worker, apparently charged with keeping me from lapsing into hysterics. She asked me who she should call, and I gave her the phone numbers of my sister Mary Beth and our minister Rev. Pam Fickenscher. Soon both of them—my sister still wearing her swimsuit coverup—were sitting with me in the waiting room.

Another hour or two passed, and the doctor returned. "We weren't able to extract the clot," he said. "The next few days will be critical as we see how his brain responds. Swelling is our biggest fear. He is unconscious, but our CT and MRI scans show that a large part of the left side of his brain has been destroyed. The left side controls the right side of his body, his speech and language, and some executive function. We've moved him upstairs into the Neuro ICU. You can see him soon."

I tried to rise, but my legs no longer seemed to work. I burst into tears, babbling about my mom, my trip, my phone—guilt and grief overtaking me. Rob's brain—home to his endless creativity, his humor, his impressive organizational skills, his warmth, his patience, his love—what had happened to that big, beautiful brain? Would it ever be the same again? Would it ever come close? Would I still know the husband who was left?

In those first hours I was not strong or stoic or anything a middle-aged Midwestern woman should be. Instead, I wept and wailed and threw myself on my sister, my minister, even on a strange social worker. I couldn't imagine what might come next. I couldn't bear to.

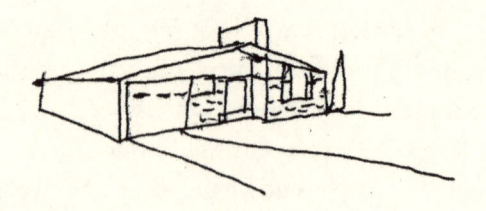

BEFORE: ROB

I have always lived big and messy. My underwear drawer looks like a hurricane hit it, and for many years my datebook consisted of a giant desktop calendar on which I scrawled appointments and reminders in a crazy fashion. I needed my schedule right in front of me, and I needed lots of room for my life. I was in a hurry, often haphazard, and my calendar showed it.

Rob, on the other hand, always so much more careful and contained, relied on pocket-sized Mead Week-at-a-Glance calendars—a tiny line for each hour of the workday and an even slimmer one for evening appointments.

A few months after his stroke, I found Rob's final datebook in his desk drawer. In the lines of his pocket calendar, the great demands on his time become so awfully apparent. It contained his whole big, sprawling life. In it you could find—painstakingly written in a miniaturized version of the block lettering peculiar to his profession—each client meeting, design session, dental appointment, and fourth-grade field trip, every letter and word perfectly placed on the lines.

Here is the Monday before his stroke:

<u>JULY 10</u>
6:15–7:15 A.M. NICHOLSON
8 A.M. PICK UP CAR
BANK
10 OSTBY, FUNK/POST, HU, MADSON
11 PETERSON
NOON SWIM
1 MAKE DINNER
2–4 PETERSON
4 JOURNAL
5 GERLOFF/LAMB (OUR KITCHEN PLAN)

Later in the week, he had made notations that I was visiting my parents, that he must take Grace to a violin lesson, an orthodontist appointment, and a friend's house, and Julia to speech class.

His life was laid out on a collection of faint lines, so full of clients and family and friends, along with his earnest attempts to exercise, read, write, and think about architecture. Was it all too much for him? Should I have seen the pressure on Rob and tried to ease it? Did his busy schedule contribute to his stroke, as one blunt neighbor had wondered aloud to me?

Rob knew from the early days of our parenthood that I needed to work, have breaks, go out with friends. In other words, I needed a full partner in parenthood. Loving children, adoring our particular two children, he quickly and happily dove into the breach. From the first, he brought the girls along as he did projects about the house. "What doin', Dad?" became toddler Grace's most frequent remark as together they repaired window screens or changed lightbulbs.

In my more rational moments, I understood what the doctors had told me: that Rob's stroke was caused by a spontaneous dissection of his carotid artery—an inherent weakness in his vascular system. But I couldn't help but wonder if the pressures of his jam-packed life had contributed to the pressure in his veins.

In my less rational moments, as I struggled to sleep, I wondered if I could have done more to erase a few of those calendar entries, thus easing some of the terrible weight from his body and life.

The organization and attention to detail exhibited by Rob's calendar characterized his entire life. As for architecture, he had known since age 7 that he wanted to pursue that career. Inspired by his own family's architect-designed mid-century modern home, Rob started sketching floor plans as a grade schooler, began working as a draftsman in high school, and entered architecture school as an undergraduate.

He grew up a quiet, bookish child, with one much older sister. His father was a botany professor, warm, effusive, and outdoorsy, always taking the family on backpacking or canoe trips. His mother was quiet, artistic, elegant, an introverted reader. She encouraged Rob's interests in reading, photography, and architecture, but was not overly invested in parenting, which suited Rob just fine. By junior high he was riding his bike all over his hometown of Madison and far into the countryside beyond, reading constantly, and learning to take and develop professional-looking photographs. By high school he was spending most of his time at home in his room.

By the time I met him when he was 31, Rob had a large, carefully chosen library that covered several walls of his apartment. He methodically organized his books by subject—artists, architects, history, design—and alphabetically within each topic. Woe to the careless friend who shoved a book about Frank Lloyd Wright into the Bauhaus section.

After his stroke, I looked through Rob's computer desktop. On it I found a list of design and development essay ideas for the neighborhood newspaper, computer renderings of nearly a dozen projects, letters to his friends and his parents. Above his desk was tacked Julia's drawing of her dad, complete with round glasses and receding hairline, and next to it, a photo of Rob with his arms around both girls, sitting on the lakeside dock near our home. Lake Harriet, just blocks away, was the near nightly destination for our foursome. First, a ride on the trolley; then a short stroll down the hill to feed the ducks and buy popcorn and ice cream.

Upstairs, inside Rob's top dresser drawer, was a photo-ready display of perfectly folded T-shirts, shorts, and socks, one color each. By his bedside was a small table pure in its simplicity, holding just a book, a pen, a cup.

The sanctity of our bedroom was absolute. For Rob it represented a fiercely defended oasis of organization and calm set within a storm of family chaos—recipe books, school permission slips, Barbie dolls, teapots, stuffed pandas, bike helmets—which constantly threatened to engulf our small house.

Rob loved to travel. He had once spent a month in Finland studying the work of Alvar Aalto and had crisscrossed Europe several times. He loved to cross-country ski, kayak, hike, and bicycle. He tried his best to cook.

Although I can no longer hear it in my head, Rob once possessed a warm, soft, fluid voice. Sometimes I can still detect its echoes in his laugh. Rob was articulate, passionate about the importance of home and place, dauntingly intelligent, intimidatingly well read.

By age 45, he had accomplished and learned more than most people do in a lifetime. He had planned to work into his nineties, as two of his architectural heroes, Frank Lloyd Wright and Philip Johnson, had done. He was really only beginning his career when his body forced him to end it. One key artery, the carotid, in what doctors later speculated was a genetically weak circulatory system, failed him, and his entire rich and promising life came to a sudden halt.

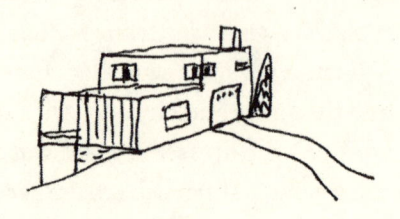

BEFORE: LYNETTE

I spent the second half of my childhood in Madison, the same city where Rob grew up. Like Rob, I was a university brat, though my dad was an administrator rather than a professor. In our house, music lessons, foreign languages, gourmet cooking, traveling, and excelling in school were emphasized. Four years older than he, I didn't meet Robert in Madison; he was the age of my younger sister, Mary Beth. We met many years later, both of us single professionals living in Minneapolis.

I was in as much of a hurry to start my work life as he had been, in my case a journalism career I had focused on since high school. In my early twenties, I was briefly and disastrously married, then had a seven-year relationship with a fun but commitment averse guy.

When I met Rob, I was working at my dream job as managing editor of *Utne Reader* magazine. A digest of the alternative press, *Utne Reader* had exploded in circulation and fame in the years since I began working there, going from 75,000 to 300,000 readers and being featured in movies and furniture stores. I loved poring over books and articles to find the best and most interesting readings to publish. I enjoyed the attention and travel that working there brought me, but mostly I adored the smart and quirky staff members, many of whom became lifelong friends. I owned my own condo, traveled as much as I could, read constantly, and enjoyed theater and films.

Unlike Rob, I was messy, extroverted, moved quickly, loved parties, struggled with my temper, neglected my car's maintenance, and was famous for my frequent, loud, infectious laugh. I had two sisters—one in the Twin Cities, one in Green Bay—and my beloved parents were still in their early sixties, living in Madison.

I had made and maintained dozens of friendships with people I'd met in grade school, high school, college, grad school, various apartment buildings, and each of the half dozen jobs I'd held since college. Life was good, but something was missing. I wanted to get married and have kids. I was 34 years old and had lived alone for eight years. I was ready.

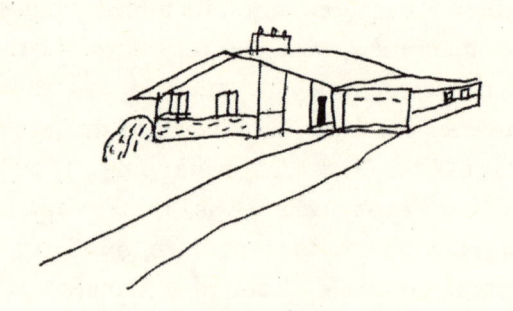

1992: MEETING AND MARRYING

About six months after I stopped seeing my elusive longtime boyfriend, I met Rob on a warm fall day. My sister Mary Beth, who'd been a classmate of his, told me he was a local architect and writer, so I hired him to write an essay for *Utne Reader*. Soon afterwards, we arranged to have lunch. At the time, he was finishing a master's degree in architecture at Virginia Tech, having only returned to Minneapolis for a visit.

My first reaction upon seeing him was, Yikes, he's short! At 5 foot 6, he was a full inch shorter than me, and I'd never liked dating small guys. But Rob had a warm smile full of huge teeth, and I knew from his writing that he was thoughtful and smart. I decided to quash my objections to his stature long enough to share lunch.

And what a lunch it was. I know we ate, but what I remember most is how easily and quickly we talked—about our idiosyncratic hometown, about writing, about our university fathers and university-wife mothers, about architecture and urban planning.

Even more remarkably, when we parted company, he said something I'd never before heard a man utter: "I feel as if I monopolized the conversation." He hadn't, of course, but that he was even aware of such a possibility put him light years ahead of most men I knew.

Six months later, in early March, by then resettled in Minneapolis, Rob invited me to his apartment for dinner. He wasn't much of a cook (the chicken was bloody, the rice hard) but once again, the food was beside the point. We had another intense conversation, a real meeting of the minds, and I suddenly found myself attracted to him as more than a friend.

All of which made me panic, say a quick goodbye, and bolt out the door.

Fortunately, that was not the end of our relationship, but the beginning. From there it went quickly: We were engaged by Memorial Day and married in a small family ceremony in late September.

At that first lunch, Rob and I began a conversation—a friendship—that would remain at the core of our relationship. Ours was never a passionate physical affair, an athletic companionship, or a merging of shared hobbies. Instead, it was a marriage based on language: reading and writing and talking about everything from the latest *New Yorker* article to the mysteries of why our daughters refused to fall asleep. We talked and talked and talked. Until, suddenly, we no longer could.

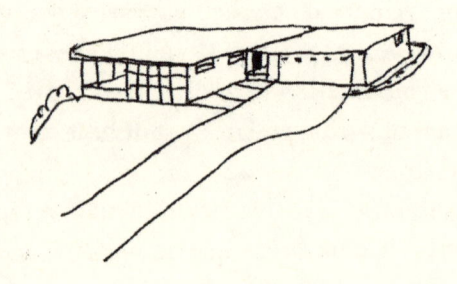

THE ICU

That first night, I set up camp in the ICU waiting room with Mary Beth. The room was windowless and dim, furnished with ugly institutional floral furniture and a scattering of sturdy end tables.

If any other frantic families shared the space with us, I cannot recall them now. Mary Beth contacted a few of my friends, and soon they began showing up with snacks and drinks, blankets and pillows. Eventually, with the help of an Ambien, I drifted into a few hours of restless sleep.

That first night would be the only one I spent at the hospital. I know many stroke wives never leave their husband's bedsides, but I decided that the two small girls at home needed me more. I couldn't leave Grace and Julia—still anxiously attached to us following their adoptions from China as toddlers—under the care of even the kindest relatives.

But that first week I did spend most of my daytime hours in the ICU, especially the first two days, when the doctors' pronouncements were unrelentingly grim. Here's what came at me during those initial 48 hours: "He might not make it. The next few days are critical. If he does survive, he will probably spend his life in a nursing home. The brain damage is extensive. Most stroke victims' brains swell catastrophically. If that happens, you'll have some hard decisions to make."

How could Rob go in one day from redesigning our kitchen and taking our daughters on trolley rides to lying inert and unconscious in an ICU bed, the doctors predicting his death?

DAY 2

The morning after Rob's stroke, I woke up in the waiting room and remembered that he was hovering near death. My stomach lurched. The first thing Mary Beth told me was that Rob's mother, Mary Ellen, had arrived late the previous night. This did not comfort me as the arrival of my own mother would have done. Mary Ellen—known by her grandchildren as Mimi—was a tidy woman of 80, perfectly coiffed and usually dressed in jewel-toned separates and matching jewelry. Frosty and prim, she always made me feel like a giant, messy goofball, my jokes and loud laugh unwelcome interruptions in her quiet family home. But we both adored her son, so I hoped her presence would be reassuring to Rob.

Those hopes were dashed the instant she walked in. Mimi's first words were not to ask about Rob but to complain about the discomfort of her hospital cot. A flash of anger shot through me: was that *really* the most important issue right now? Weeks later I learned that Mary Beth had to work hard to persuade

Mimi into making the trip to Minneapolis; she hadn't thought it necessary.

We found Rob unconscious in the ICU, every part of his body hooked up to tubes and wires. The doctors weren't optimistic about his chances. The MRI scans, they told us, showed a lot of damage to his brain.

Soon the doctors and social workers had whisked me, Mimi, and Rob's closest childhood friend, Karen (the daughter of a neurologist), into a conference room to discuss the tough stuff. The biggest danger in the next three days, they told us, was that Rob's assaulted brain would swell dangerously against his skull, putting deadly pressure on it. If that happened, we had to make a choice: Should the surgeons remove the top of Rob's skull, thus allowing his brain to swell unimpeded, or should we let nature take its course?

Mimi said, "I think Rob would rather die than live with serious brain damage. Being an architect is so important to him. I don't think he would want the surgery." I understood her point—indeed Rob had even signed a health care directive asking that no extreme measures be taken to keep him alive—but what was once a theoretical decision was now an actual one, and the stakes were much higher. Mostly I was thinking of our girls, who had already lost their birth parents. Could I really let their beloved father slip away without a fight? In the end, when faced with this life-or-death decision, my answer contradicted Mimi's: I told the doctors that if Rob's brain swelled, they should perform the surgery and try to save his life.

Of course, making this decision didn't mean I was some self-sacrificing paragon of womanhood. I dreaded the prospect of a damaged spouse. I was an unlikely candidate for the job of devoted caregiver—impatient, social, independent, and easily frustrated. For nine years I had counted on Rob to provide me with regular breaks from the house and the kids. Now those days were over.

But to give up on him entirely—to not even *try* to save him—was unthinkable. I kept imagining Grace and Julia's reactions. They were devoted to their dad, who often had more patience and energy for them than I did. He took them canoeing and bicycling; he read to them for hours. He patiently drove them hundreds of miles over several steamy July days so the girls could visit all the sites on a Laura Ingalls Wilder pilgrimage to Walnut Grove and DeSmet, even happily agreeing to don an 1870s outfit last seen on Pa Ingalls. What would they do without him?

Regardless of what his altered mental status meant for me or for his mother, I knew our daughters would prefer to have a cognitively compromised father than none at all. So, to the gathering of people in that hospital conference room, I squeaked out once again, "We want him around. We want the surgery."

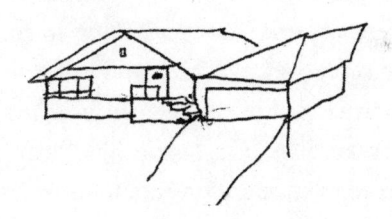

THREE POLAROIDS

The only photos I have from those first terrible days Rob spent in the ICU are three Polaroids. For some reason, a nurse insisted on taking them, and all these years later, I am glad she did.

Two are nearly identical: Rob tethered to multiple tubes and hoses, his eyes closed, utterly still, lying on his side in a bed with bumpers not unlike those on a baby's crib. And then one photo taken perhaps a day later, the girls and me standing next to Rob's bed. By then his eyes were half open, and he was trying to look into the camera. In this picture, I held onto Grace; she and I were both smiling dutifully for the camera.

What haunts me is the image of Julia, who was standing between us and her devastated Dad. The look on her face was so full of sadness, loss, confusion, and grief that I can barely glance at it all these years later.

Julia was just 6 when the father she had known, loved, and counted on—the man who flew to China to bring her home, whom she clung to for many weeks afterwards—was no longer accessible to her. He couldn't move or speak. Her terror centered on a blue oxygen plug lodged inside his nostril. It made Rob look foreign to her and seemed to represent everything that had changed about him.

His strange appearance was compounded a day later when an overly efficient orderly—not bothering to consult the family photos in the room, all of which showed Rob with a beard—shaved his jaw. Julia had never seen him without a beard and Grace and I had seen him so just once. The clean-shaven man in the ICU bed looked even more foreign to us now.

When I think back on the days when Rob was unconscious and unable to respond, it feels as if they lasted for weeks. But when I re-read the CaringBridge site I wrote—my own words—I realize that by the fifth day after his stroke, Rob was already touching us and even goofing around with some small stuffed animals the girls had brought in, pushing the toys' plush noses into the girls' noses; dancing the tiny bears across his bed. In

CaringBridge I wrote, "They glowed from having some interaction again with their Dad."

I visited Robert every one of the ten days he spent in the hospital, but I did not camp out in his room as so many spouses do. Instead, I passed most of my time at home with the girls. Our 20-year-old nanny, Heidi, was there, too. Friends rallied around to take the girls on overnights, outings, and playdates.

And every night I put the girls to bed, lying with each one in turn, reading to them and staying in their beds until they fell asleep. "Dad's going to be okay," I would say to Julia, trying to open a conversation about the topic that I knew terrified her. "The doctors say he will be home in a couple of months, after he learns to walk again." "Can we have more ice cream cups when we see Dad tomorrow?" she'd ask in response.

Grace and Julia had never fallen asleep easily. They needed close contact with a parent to relax enough to drift off. Now they needed that physical and emotional reassurance from me even more. Each night I spent at least an hour on this bedtime ritual.

In the weeks and years that followed Rob's stroke, I was an imperfect mother. I periodically blew up at the girls, I took vacations alone, I could be impatient and angry. But this bedtime routine, this I did, no matter how desperately I wanted to be alone. Julia and I—tucked in tight with a dozen stuffed animals in her bed beneath the eaves—read and re-read a whimsical book about a snowman visited by woodland animals called *The Stranger in the Woods*. Grace and I finished the Harry Potter series she and her dad had been working their way through.

I continued this bedtime ritual with Grace for about a year after Rob's stroke. Once she hit 11, she could calm herself at night, often re-reading the Harry Potter books her father had once read to her.

But for Julia, my tenderhearted younger child, that need for evening comfort from Mom would last far longer, and she remained a steadfast homebody until she left for college.

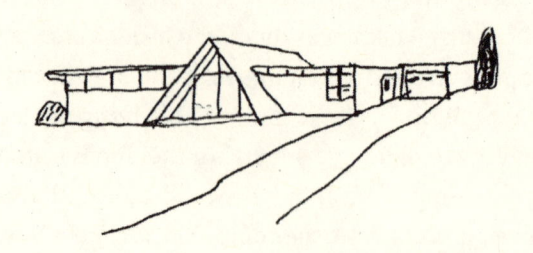

FRIENDS AND PROGRESS

Over those first two days while Rob remained unconscious and the outlook for his future appeared bleak, dozens of our friends rushed in, surrounding us with love in the sterile hallways of Fairview Southdale Hospital.

Doug, a Delta Airlines pilot, visited while still in uniform. Heidi, whose own husband had died of a heart attack the previous year, flew from Phoenix to comfort us. When I saw David D., Rob's closest friend from architecture school, I threw myself into his arms, crying, "They say he's going to die!" David, who had first known Rob as an intense and talented 20-year-old, looked back at me, his face contorted by grief.

On Tuesday night, to the amazement of Rob's medical team, he regained consciousness and showed us that he could hear us and understand at least some of what was going on.

The next day, Rob's neurologist, Dr. Bruce Idelkope, told me that neural imaging had shown many small capillaries in Rob's brain were reconnecting, bringing blood to his brain's damaged left hemisphere. As we held our collective breath over the next few days, Rob's big, beautiful brain, which had survived such a grievous insult, never showed signs of the predicted and potentially deadly swelling.

The neurological damage was extensive, of course, and the rehab road ahead would be a long one. But Rob was going to live and learn. At that moment, it seemed like enough.

One aspect of Rob's increasing awareness took me by surprise. I had placed family photos around his hospital room, and on day five, he began gesturing toward a photo of his parents, pointing at his father, Jerry, who had been dead for five years. He repeatedly stabbed a finger toward the photo and then sketched a shrug that I knew meant: What gives? I suddenly realized that Rob was asking me why his father hadn't visited him in the hospital. Rob had forgotten everything about Jerry's long decline and death; he remembered only his father's consistent, lifelong warmth and love.

So it was that Rob had to learn all over again that his beloved father was gone. When I told him, as gently as I could, tears spilled from his eyes.

THREE BOOKS

Three books, each distressing in its own way, stick in my mind from the two weeks Rob spent in the ICU.

The first was a mystery my then-brother-in-law Rick brought Rob as a gift. This present so clearly demonstrated the utter cluelessness or denial most of our family and friends were living in during those early weeks. Rob could barely stay awake and was incapable of understanding or expressing language. How was he supposed to read a complicated mystery set in New Orleans? Yet for weeks that stupid book sat on Rob's bedside table, a cruel reminder of both the stroke's toll and our loved ones' incomprehension of its devastation.

The second book was sent to me by well-meaning friends, its title something like *How to be the Most Selfless Caretaker Ever*. It was essentially a guidebook for how the reader (a woman, of course) should harness all her energy and her best self in order to martyr herself for her ill spouse—and to do so happily. It promised that route would lead to the caretaker's ultimate spiritual triumph.

That book particularly enraged me. Apparently, it wasn't enough that I was handling a full-time job, an architectural practice, two distraught girls, a house, health care and insurance paperwork, and daily consultations with doctors, therapists, and friends—now I must also plan to devote my life to caretaking? And to do so in a cheerful, even saintly fashion? No thanks.

I tossed that book in the garbage soon after it arrived.

The third book was a giant three-ring binder, a handbook covering every last depressing detail about strokes. This, of course, was thrust upon me by an energetic hospital social worker. Ever the obedient student, I began paging through the giant binder but soon became overwhelmed. So, I stuck this handbook into the bookcase and steadfastly ignored it. Of course, every time I spied it there, I felt guilty, as if I were skipping the required reading. Finally, about a year later, I tossed this book, too. Who can possibly take in this difficult information—all at once—while still reeling from your spouse's stroke and just trying to get through one day at a time?

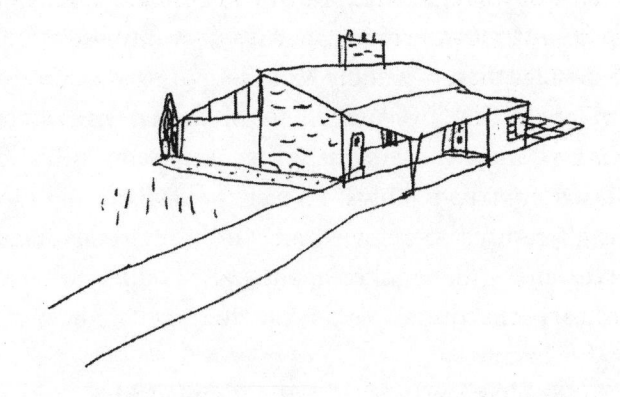

CARINGBRIDGE

My regular habit in the weeks following Rob's stroke was to retreat into his office. Located in a separate building attached to our garage, his office was where all our computers were kept, and where some bit of peace resided for me, away from the girls, the nannies, and the friends helping us with laundry and meals.

A couple of our closest friends started a CaringBridge blog for us a few days after Rob's stroke. I had never heard of CaringBridge, but it soon proved to be an invaluable way to keep friends and family updated on Rob's condition without fielding dozens of emails and phone calls.

By day five I had taken over the blog, employing my best writing skills to provide mostly upbeat posts on Rob's condition and location, visits from family and friends, and other news. I typically ended each entry with a long list of thank yous to all the people who were helping us out.

My tone was positive, funny, optimistic—pretty much the opposite of the way I felt at the time. I'm not sure why I wasn't more honest in my writing, but it's probably because I've always dreaded pity. When my Mom fought breast cancer, when I divorced my first husband, when I struggled with infertility—through all these earlier times of fear and sadness, I had rarely shown my true feelings. I never spoke about my mother's cancer, I refused to return home for Christmas during my divorce, and I made jokes about my inability to conceive—once nearly shutting down a book club meeting by describing myself as barren.

Two weeks after Rob's stroke, I wrote a chirpy entry about the beauty of his "large, private room with a treetop view" at the acute rehab center, blathering on about the facility's therapeutic pool, "nice-sized dining room," large lounge, outdoor patio, etc. It sounded like a travel brochure for a desirable beach resort.

My actual response to touring the rehabilitation center was to sink into a mini-depression. I first toured the place with Mimi, and as we walked the halls, we saw people slumped over in wheelchairs and gimping along the corridors. Dozens of men and women, many of them younger than Rob, unable to speak, eat solid food, or use their arms and legs. This acute rehab center, despite its flower-filled patio and brightly colored artwork, was every bit an institution—an institution where I knew Rob must live for weeks.

Yes, my brilliant, once-active husband would now spend his days and nights in this despair-filled place, trying to remember how to swallow and to distinguish *yes* from *no*. When we finished the tour, I felt a familiar lump rising in my throat and knew I would cry if I spoke. Mimi, on the other hand, seemed pleased with the place. "Well," she said cheerfully, "this is very nice." Desperate to make her understand my feelings, I said, "I just never expected the 'in sickness and in health' part to kick in so soon." "Hmmm," was her reply.

So back I went to CaringBridge, writing cheerfully about the friend who brought his oil paintings to Rob's room or the time we snuck in our cats. What I was really thinking was, Help me, somebody. I'm drowning and I'm terrified. But I couldn't stand to be so vulnerable in print, in front of so many people. Not yet, at least, and not for many years to come.

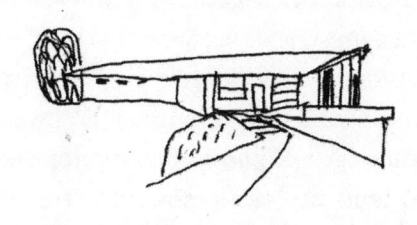

SISTER KENNY

When someone, especially someone young like Rob, has a stroke, there are so many questions about the future. Will he walk again? Talk again? Will he regain the use of his right arm and hand? Will he read? Return to work? All these questions played on repeat through my head like some unholy chorus.

Of course, our friends and family were firing the same questions at me, and as fast as they could ask, I deflected them through the distancing device of my cheerful CaringBridge site, saving my pain for the privacy of my room.

For those first few awful days it had looked as if Rob might never live at home again, much less read *The New Yorker*. The neurologist just shook his head at the MRI scans, looking sadly at the giant blank spaces where the blood clot, unchecked, had done its awful work. "I think you had better prepare yourself to move him to a nursing home," he told me. The thought of Rob, 45, stuck in some depressing institution with drooling 90-year-olds filled me with horror.

But the neurologist, happily, was wrong in his catastrophizing, and only two weeks after Rob's stroke, we moved him into an acute rehab center called Sister Kenny Institute, attached to Abbott Northwestern Hospital in Minneapolis. There he received twice daily physical, occupational, and speech therapy, and there it was that I allowed myself to hope again.

Sister Kenny was named for the polio nurse who made it famous a century earlier. Rob spent a month there, learning to walk, swallow food, and dress himself again. The girls and I, often accompanied by a nanny, visited him every evening after dinner.

Because it was summer and the weather was sunny and warm, we usually wheeled Rob up to the second-floor patio, which featured a few flowerpots and an old glider that the girls loved to swing on.

Back in those early days, Rob couldn't speak except to say hello, but he often hummed "Hail to the Chief" or "Happy Birthday" as we rolled him outside. His smile was always huge when he spied us coming down the hallway.

The girls quickly became accustomed to the place, raiding the fridge for cups of cranberry juice and crushed ice, running down the hallways, playing with their Barbies and even—in one unintended bit of black humor—pretending the busty dolls were having strokes. Sometimes we even snuck our small cats Kit and Angel into his room, and seeing their fuzzy yellow faces always lit up his. As he reached out his left hand toward them and dropped his cheek onto their soft fur you could see his whole body relax.

Like most hospital rooms, Rob's was full of ugly, clunky oak furniture and featured a view of a parking ramp. In other words, his 12- by 14-foot world was depressing, especially for an architect so sensitive to the space around him, so we escaped to the patio whenever possible. The fresh air was a reprieve for us all, though it was impossible to forget for a minute where we were.

Just two months earlier, Rob had been taking Julia and Grace for rides on the Lake Harriet trolley or walking them to archery practice at Lake Bde Maka Ska. He had been rushing out to his backyard office every morning at 6, eager to get in a few hours of sketching before the phones started ringing and the daily deluge began.

Now he was confined to a wheelchair, unable to speak, read, or write, mute and paralyzed, his life's work having shrunk down to daily attempts to swallow solid foods and use his legs.

Most days in this new life, Rob and I put our heads down and muscled through the tasks set before us: for him, dressing himself with one hand or pronouncing his daughters' names, for me, navigating disability insurance paperwork or attending back-to-school picnics.

But sometimes, especially late at night when sleep wouldn't come, the fears, regrets, and overwhelming loss of the past few months threatened to swamp me.

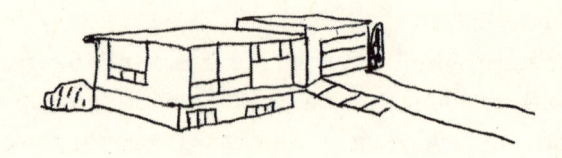

FORK, COMB, KEY

August was in full steamy swing when I stopped by Sister Kenny one morning to accompany Rob to speech therapy. By now he had been living at the rehab center for two weeks, receiving daily physical, occupational, and speech therapy, as well as occasional—if not always well received—sessions of music, acupuncture, and other nontraditional therapies.

But of all those efforts toward recovery, speech therapy loomed the largest. Learning to talk again was the most important thing in the world to Rob (and to me), and I knew he worked hard at it daily. But I couldn't help but wonder what exactly Rob did with his speech therapist, given that he still had trouble understanding most conversation and his vocabulary was stalled at two words: *baby* and *bible*. (Incidentally, because automatic speech, which comes from the right brain, is the first to reappear, most people with strokes start by blurting out swear words. Certainly, if I had been the stroke victim, the air around me would have turned blue. It was typical of my sweet-natured husband that his early vocabulary was so pure.)

Rob's speech therapist made a point of asking me to attend his next session, and I was nothing if not dutiful. And curious. I pushed Rob's wheelchair down the beige hallways to the tiny, windowless room that served as his therapist's office. As we arrived, I wondered, as always, how much more therapeutic a beautifully designed space might be—for any patient, but especially for an architect like Rob, so aware of his surroundings. I was certain that every day he spent in this colorless, institutional space crushed his soul a little.

But the design details of the Sister Kenny rehab center weren't the most pressing matter at hand. Mentally shaking myself, I redirected my attention to the painfully earnest speech therapist facing us across the desk.

What transpired next was probably the most excruciating 30 minutes of my life. I can't remember what the speech therapist said; indeed, I can't even remember her name. But I will never forget the exercise she set forth for Rob that day.

On the desk between herself and Rob she placed a fork, a key, a comb, a hammer, and a pen. She didn't ask him to come up with the names of these items or pronounce them; she asked only that he point to each one in turn as she named it.

Which he was unable to do.

To sit there and watch my brilliant husband flummoxed by the task of distinguishing a fork from a pen was the lowest point of the stroke odyssey for me—and probably for him.

The desolation I'd been running from for weeks overwhelmed me. Caring for the girls, filing paperwork, making daily hospital visits, writing the CaringBridge blog—these tasks had been my frantic armor against despair. But here in this colorless shoebox, I confronted the enormity of all that Rob had lost. And what I had lost as well.

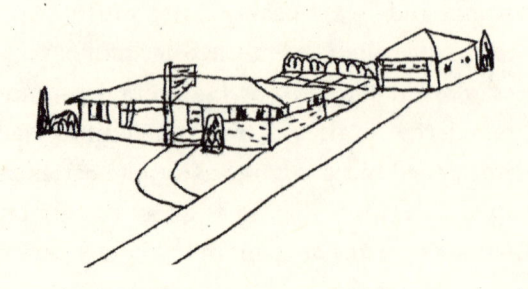

WHAT THE FUTURE HOLDS

One evening, about two weeks into Rob's monthlong stay at Sister Kenny, his physiatrist, Dr. Barbara Seizert, took me by the arm and moved me into a quiet corner. I asked her, "How is Rob doing? What does his future look like?" And she stared me straight in the eye and said, "Lynette, professionals who suffer major left-brain strokes almost never return to work. You need to know that."

I stood there gaping at her. Aren't doctors supposed to hold out hope for their patients and families? Aren't they meant to urge us on, to try harder and work more? I thought about Pastor Warren, who had returned to work as a minister, and of actress Patricia Neal, who had famously returned to work on stage and screen. If they could do it, why couldn't Rob?

He couldn't do it, not for lack of will or effort, but because these examples are the exceptions, not the rule.

Dr. Seizert repeated her message, as if to ensure that it had truly sunk in. It had. I felt like she had punched me in the stomach. As we stood there together in silence, I thought of everything her prediction meant for Robert. No more designing beautiful houses or producing plan books or writing articles about urbanism. His career was over.

But even as I stood there, crushed by grief, I felt the truth of her words, along with a sliver of relief. There would be no ambivalence about this part of our future, at least. When it came to Robert Gerloff Residential Architects, I knew what must be done.

My first job was to convince Rob's young associate, Jeremiah Battles—who kept asking me when Rob would be returning to the office—that his boss would never work again and that we would be closing his office. Jeremiah needed to farm out all the design projects that had just been started and finish those that were nearer completion.

Over the next few months, together we would wrap up the work of Robert Gerloff Residential Architects, housed in the cozy backyard office Rob had designed just seven years earlier. By the time the new year rolled around, we would close that office door for good, shutting down Rob's lifelong dreams with it.

If I had it to do over again, I would have taken Rob out to his office and we would have reviewed the magical work he had created in 20 years of practice. Together we would have pored over the photos and blueprints of the many light-filled kitchens and breezy porches he had designed over the years. We would have held a closing ceremony with the girls, Jeremiah, and perhaps a few favorite clients. We would have marked and honored the end of an era.

But we never did; I never even thought of it. Instead, as the years went by, Rob's office slowly became a place for suitcase storage, preteen sleepovers, and Christmas present wrapping.

Later, when we decided to move into an apartment, we sold his entire architectural library to a used bookstore and tossed his client blueprints and files into a dumpster.

We cleaned and pitched and sorted until finally all that was left of that office, designed and built with such hope and happiness, was the memory of a man who had arrived at his vocation as a 7-year-old boy and had followed that path with unwavering energy and joy until a single blood clot closed off every possibility of architecture except for the love of it.

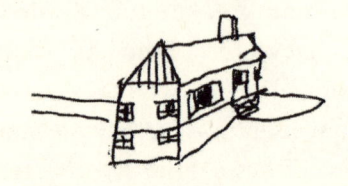

COURAGE CENTER

Moving Rob to Courage Center in early September felt like real progress. For one thing, it was a rehab facility not attached to a hospital, meaning that his medical condition was considered stable. For another, it had an idyllic suburban setting, placed on a stream and surrounded by gardens, each room offering a peaceful view. Finally, this place was famous for the physical progress its patients made. Within a few days, the therapists assured me that by the time Rob came home he would be walking—and not just walking but climbing stairs and dressing himself.

The girls and I continued our visits each evening, but at least at Courage Center we could burst fully into the outdoors and into the beautiful late summer and early fall Minnesota evenings, Grace and Julia vying to push Rob's wheelchair along the creek. Often Julia would hop on his lap and Grace would push them fast down the pathways. They always hoped to spy the great white egret who lived there, whom they had rather uncreatively named Whitey.

Then there were ice chips to locate and snacks to snatch up, and the cards and gifts to review that Rob's visitors had left during the day.

Sometimes I also visited Rob in the mornings, watching as he worked with the physical therapists teaching him how to walk, the occupational therapists teaching him to work in the kitchen, and the speech therapists helping him to talk again. It was the speech therapists who had the really heavy lifting, since Rob's aphasia (the loss of the ability to understand or express speech) proved to be the most persistent part of his disability.

Later I would learn that Courage Center therapists were some of the youngest and most inexperienced in town, since the jobs didn't pay well. This proved especially problematic for speech therapy, where practice working with stroke survivors makes all the difference. His lack of progress in that area discouraged us both.

Despite that, we were lucky that Rob could spend two months at Courage Center. That extra time in rehab allowed him to come home mostly independent, unlike the husbands of so many of my stroke friends, who still needed help showering and dressing for months after returning home. In this we were assisted by the roll of the dice that is American health care. Rob had purchased top-of-the-line health insurance for his small business, and it ended up covering almost every dollar of the ridiculously high bills he racked up during his recovery.

Years later for a class, Rob wrote about his time living at Courage Center, and I found it moving to read what he remembered most:

> AFTER HAVING MY STROKE, I SPENT ABOUT TWO MONTHS CALLED COURAGE CENTER. IT WAS WONDERFUL BECAUSE IT HAD LOTS OF FREEDOM, AND I COULD LOOK FOR THE BIRDS IN THE POND. LYNETTE, GRACE, AND JULIA VISITED ME IN THE EVENING, AND WHILE GRACE WAS SITTING ON MY LAP IN MY WHEELCHAIR AND JULIA WAS PUSHING ME TOWARD THE POND: WE LOOKED FOR THE GREAT BLUE HERON, OR THE GREAT EGRET OUTSIDE, AND A COOT AND MALLARD DUCK. SOMETIMES WE WOULDN'T SEE ANY BIRDS.
>
> I FRANTICALLY WOULD WORK HARD AND A GUY WOULD PUSH ME IN MY WHEELCHAIR AT PT AND OT. AND SPEECH THERAPY AND I COULD SEE A LOT OF STROKE FROM THE LAST MONTH AND I COULD SEE THERE WERE TWO STROKES: ONE, THEY WERE WORKING VERY HARD AND TWO, THEY GAVE IT UP. I WAS HORRIFIED AND WOULD NEVER QUIT.

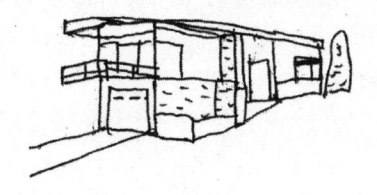

NEUROPSYCHOLOGICAL EXAM

Just before Rob came home, a neuropsychologist did a thorough evaluation of his neurological condition. I don't remember reading it closely at the time, which was probably for the best. Because when I recently reviewed its findings, they were discouraging. Dr. Jacalyn Kawiecki noted that "it is difficult to assess the client because of his deep expressive aphasia." Meaning he couldn't talk at all.

At this point Rob was routinely saying *yes* when he meant *no*, and vice versa. He couldn't tell her with any certainty whether he was left- or right-handed. She noted that "the client has profound receptive language deficits." Meaning he didn't comprehend a thing she said.

Dr. Kawiecki did have more luck, as the girls and I did, with getting Rob to understand things by miming them or pointing to them. She also recognized that Rob wasn't "grossly depressed" and "was able to laugh and joke." Both encouraging findings, given the state he found himself in.

Rob was impulsive, the doctor noted—which I later learned was common among brain damage victims—but showed the ability to learn from experience. He also demonstrated great strength on visuospatial tasks (no surprise, given his profession) but struggled mightily with any tasks involving linguistic components. She ended her 12-page report: "The client is still grossly disabled by his stroke . . . I believe the prognosis for Mr. Gerloff's future is clouded."

MORE PROGRESS

During his three months at the Sister Kenny and Courage Center rehab facilities, Rob learned to walk again. I watched as, over the weeks, he got stronger and faster. This triumph cannot be overstated. Wheelchair bound and with a useless right side when he left the hospital, Rob could now walk—with a leg brace but no cane—and climb stairs. Thanks to regular occupational therapy, he could also shower and dress himself and prepare his own toast, cereal, and sandwiches.

The simple recitation of these accomplishment belies the weeks of hard work and pain that went into producing them. I often accompanied Rob to PT sessions, first at Sister Kenny and then in the Courage Center gym, where he struggled to walk while holding onto a double-railed path, dragging his right leg behind him. He worked hard every day and never gave up, despite daily exhaustion and frustration.

The OT sessions were easier. Perhaps because his right brain was so well developed from years of drawing and design, Rob learned to use his left hand more quickly than do most people. Soon, with the help of some handy kitchen gadgets, he was able to slice, cut, open packages and cans, dress himself, write, draw, and eat—all with his left hand.

He could even ascend and descend stairs, if there was a handrail available on both sides. Rob was ready to come home.

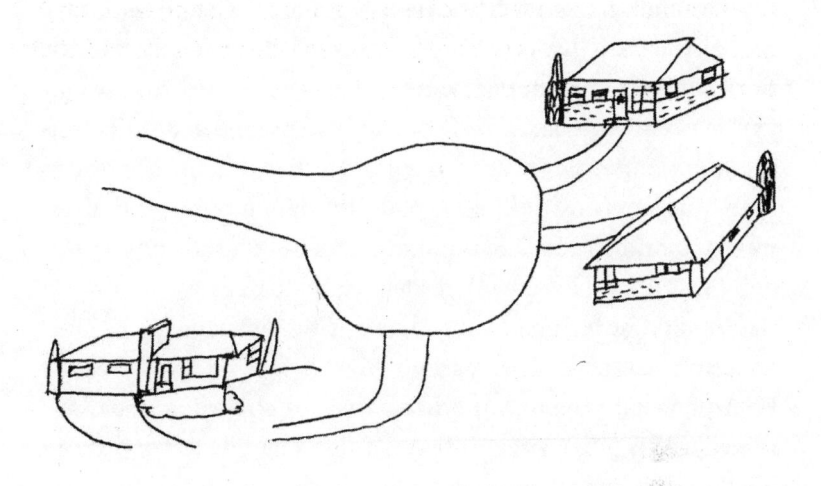

COMING HOME

At the end of October, Courage Center pronounced Robert fit to leave. It had been three and a half months since his stroke, and in that time, he had progressed from a lump in a bed to a man who could walk, climb stairs, dress and shower alone, and handle himself in the kitchen.

We had spent the intervening weeks wisely, hiring Rob's favorite contractor to install sturdy banisters along both stairways as well as adding an easily accessible shower to the first-floor bath.

Courage Center speech and occupational therapists would come to our house for the next two months to make sure Rob's progress continued, and friends were lined up to drive him to physical therapy appointments. In other words, we weren't going to be doing this alone.

Rationally, I knew the time had come for Rob to rejoin us. But emotionally I was terrified. My eyes filled with tears as the uber-competent Courage Center manager handed me two gigantic plastic pill boxes and tried to instruct me in administering their contents. I was so frightened that this frail, maimed man was now my sole responsibility. His mother and sister were 250 miles away, and our daughters were just 6 and 10 years old. I was it, and I wasn't sure I was equal to it.

What if he fell again, as he had during his first days at Courage Center, or had another seizure like the one he'd had at Sister Kenny? What if he had another stroke, or choked on food, or I mixed up his pills? What if I just couldn't handle the daily reality of caring for a disabled partner?

I wanted to tell the clinic manager that no, he wasn't ready to come home, or more to the point, I wasn't ready. I wanted Rob to stay at Courage Center, with its leafy grounds, its therapists and nursing assistants who watched over him carefully, where someone else prepared him three meals a day and monitored his pills and progress.

The girls were at school. I was back to working three days a week at Carleton College in Northfield, an hour from home. The lifeline we rented for Rob to wear around his neck—which had a button he could push if he needed immediate help—made me feel marginally better, but it didn't completely assuage my fears.

Starting today, I was the sole responsible adult in our household, charged with managing a weepy, weak stroke victim and two sad and scared grade-schoolers.

I wasn't sure I could do it. So right there, in front of the no-nonsense Courage Center manager, I burst into tears. She hugged me and told me it would all be okay, and I could call her any time.

So it was that Rob and I walked out of Courage Center and into the pale sunlight of a late fall day—and into the next part of our lives.

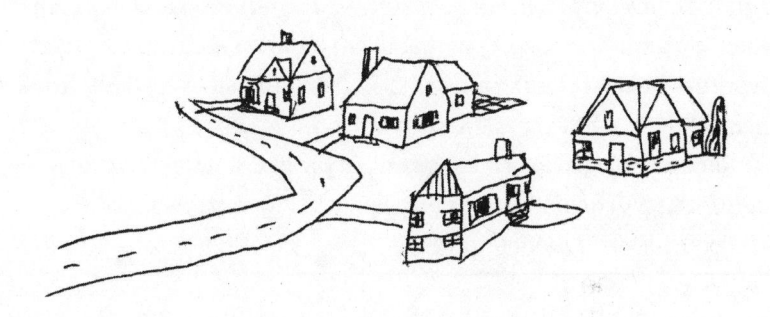

ENDING CARINGBRIDGE

I kept up the blog for another month after Rob returned home, but as Thanksgiving approached, I decided my public sharing should come to a close. I wanted to send one final message to family and friends, though, a message that would let them know in no uncertain terms that we would not be returning to our former life, but instead would be starting a new one. I wanted everyone to stop expecting our old life, especially Rob's old life, to reappear.

One of our ministers, the Rev. Pam Fickenscher, had recommended a book by Reynolds Price, who, following surgery for the spinal cancer that transformed him into a paraplegic, wrote *A Whole New Life*. His brave and honest words greatly influenced me in the weeks following Rob's stroke, so it was with those words that I concluded my final CaringBridge entry:

"Reynolds Price wrote:

Anyone who knew or loved you in your old life will be hard at work in the fierce endeavor to revive your old self, the self they recall with love or respect. Their motives are admirable...but again their care is often a brake on the way you must go. At the crucial juncture, when you turn toward the future, they'll likely have little help to offer... the kindest thing anyone could have done for me... would have been to look me squarely in the eye and say this: 'Reynolds Price is dead. Who will you be now? Who can you be and how can you get there, double-time?'

So that is Rob's task now, and mine to help him with, however I can. No, he may never again be the Rob of a million house designs, thoughtful columns, and plan books. The new Rob may be a volunteer, an even more engaged father, a gardener, a mentor—who knows?

Please stay with us on the journey, however frightening and threatening it may be. Please visit us and cheer us on. Know that we struggle with fear and self-pity too, even as we move toward embracing a whole new life."

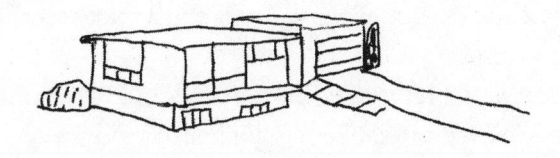

BEFORE: FUSS FACTOR FIVE

As sweet and even-tempered as Rob was, he was also an architect—a profession justifiably famous for valuing precision, a stark aesthetic, and a mania for organization.

When I first met Rob, his kitchen held four white plates, four white bowls, and two perfect glass candleholders—and that was about it. After we were married, he threw out all my tan and brown ceramic dishes (too clunky and '70s), along with my well-loved but grotty toaster oven. Then he announced that all dishes must be washed immediately after meals and he declared war on clutter.

Empty glasses must be placed immediately in the dishwasher, pillows and magazines lined up just so, beds made squarely, knickknacks eschewed. As a fairly neat person myself, this new regime didn't cause me too much trouble (except for the dish-washing edict: let them wait had always been my philosophy)—until the toddlers came along.

Toddlers are entropy machines. They love to throw blocks around the room, leave Barbie dolls in toilets, and roll crayons across the floor. The lack of order and serenity in our house drove Rob mad. The conflict between his ideal home and the messy daily reality of living with children was a recipe for tension.

Fast forward a few years, post-stroke, and life on that score had mellowed considerably. Yes, Rob still loved order, but he had a compelling reason for it now: if the left-handed scissors weren't where they were supposed to be, he couldn't open that bag of cereal. He was still frustrated by items not staying where they were intended to be kept, but his reaction was tempered by a new laid-back quality. Piles of mail he picked up without comment, dishes he washed regularly, laundry he took on himself.

As for the girls' messes (hairbrushes everywhere, rock climbing shoes and dance bags dropped by the front door, snacks left around the living room), he accepted those with equanimity. It may be a cliché to say he rarely sweated the small stuff, but it's an accurate assessment of his new personality. Today, even when the girls come home from college, tossing their coats and shoes and bags throughout the apartment, Rob just laughs and picks them up. "I love having the girls home," is all he says when confronted with the kind of mess that used to send him.

Oh, occasionally he still loses it over the tenth disappearance of his special cutting board, but these episodes are much rarer now than they'd once been.

However, one rule remains from the pre-stroke days: Stay away from his desk, and for God's sake, don't mess with his pens. They are lined up *just* so.

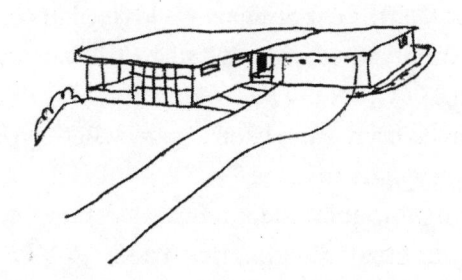

MIMI

In January 2007, a few months after Rob returned home from rehab, one of his houses was published in our local newspaper. I sent Rob's mother, Mimi, a copy, even though it depressed me just to look at it. The article's postscript informed readers that since the house had been designed, Rob had suffered a stroke and his architectural practice had closed.

By then his doctors were certain that Rob would never again work as an architect. I knew this house was the last one he would ever publish. His career, which he had loved and dreamed of since second grade, had spanned just 20 years.

Mimi seemed to share none of my bittersweet feelings, however. "Oh, how wonderful!" she trilled over the phone. "You couldn't have sent me a better gift!" Instead of her words encouraging me, as she may have intended, they made me feel more alone. The one person in the world who should have commiserated with me, the one person most likely to understand my grief over Robert's lost vocation, could not or would not acknowledge that deep loss.

A few months after the clipping incident, Mimi spent a weekend with us. That Sunday, we arrived at church early, so Rob and his mother decided to sit in the sanctuary until the service began. After only a few minutes, Mary Ellen rushed to find me. "Rob's crying and I don't know what's wrong," she said, panicked. "You *have* to come."

When I got to Rob's side, he was weeping inconsolably. In those first months following the stroke, Rob's emotions were very close to the surface ("emotionally labile," the doctors call it) and his tears, especially, were unpredictable and hard for him to control. Still, this outburst was extreme, taking place as it did in public.

Although Rob wasn't talking much at this point, I soon understood the source of his grief: he sensed that his mother was emotionally cut off from him, unwilling to really be with him in this huge loss, and her lack of support had made him cry.

I knew Mimi loved her son, but at that moment in church, struggling to comfort him, I realized that she would never walk beside us in our frightening new life. Instead, she would welcome our visits, continue her financial generosity toward our family, but studiously avoid talking about the stroke and any feelings she or we had about it.

Over the years, I tried to understand her unusual maternal response. Was Mimi's pain so great that she had to push it down rather than deal with it? Did the years she spent caring for an increasingly frail husband so deplete her that she couldn't cope with another damaged family member? Did watching her firstborn son die from a heart condition in infancy build a wall around her own heart?

Or in dealing throughout her life with a critical and domineering mother did she learn that retreat was better than engagement, withdrawal the best solution? Did she decide that it was better to protect herself rather than face her silent, disabled son?

I never learned the answers to my musings, nor did I ever untangle the mystery that was Mimi. Until her death, I scrupulously followed her unspoken rule that we would not speak of our family's greatest loss.

Years later, at Mimi's memorial service, I learned that she had spoken proudly of Rob's recovery and progress with many of her friends. Rob and I were pleased to hear that. I only wish she had told her son earlier of the pride she so readily shared with others.

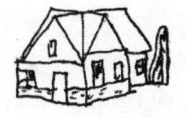

MOM

After a couple of false starts, I found a therapist I liked who specialized in grief. During the weekly wailing sessions that passed for our therapy visits, I cried as much for my mother as I did for my husband. In one of life's unfair conjunctions, my mom—a breast cancer survivor—was diagnosed with stage-four lung cancer just days before Rob's stroke. The doctors told her it was likely a consequence of the crude radiation she'd been blasted with three decades earlier during breast cancer treatment. Her prognosis was not good.

    I loved both my parents, but I had always been closer with my mom. Although she was an introvert, we were alike in so many other ways—both of us readers and writers and cooks and volunteers. Between us was a sympathy of understanding that defied language. Marjorie Anna Brehm Lamb was a warm, highly intelligent, and deeply kind woman, tall and slim, and always neatly and modestly dressed. Little makeup, little jewelry, rarely wearing new clothes, at times my mother reminded me of the nuns who had raised her from age 13 on. She took in our friends for the summers when they found themselves between apartments, regularly opened our home for large dinner parties and get-togethers, and was endlessly hospitable to her friends and ours.

    A newspaper editor when she met my father, she reluctantly gave up her career—deferring to his wishes and the standards of the times—to stay home with her three daughters. But her energy wasn't wasted. Over the years she volunteered at her churches, our schools, for a city meal program, and a local food shelf.

    All my friends adored her and blossomed in the warmth of her genuine interest and affection, and Rob was one of her biggest fans. He had designed a retirement home for my parents just 10 years earlier, a home filled with sunshine that my mother loved.

    To lose my mom just when I needed her most was among the most painful parts of Rob's stroke for me. Later my therapist would point out that I had simultaneously lost the two most important people in my life, the people who understood and loved me best. Without my life's anchors, I felt adrift.

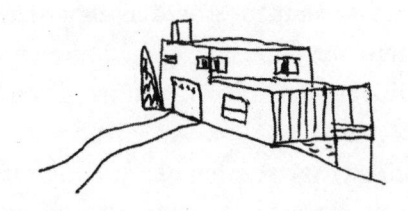

STRUGGLING WITH THE FUTURE

About a year after Rob's stroke, at the urging of a friend, I signed us up for a weekend-long stroke couples camp in western Wisconsin. It was supposed to be a combination of recreation and information, highly recommended by my friend Barb, whose husband was also a stroke survivor.

Mostly what I remember of that weekend was the cabin—which, with its single bathroom and multiple bunkbeds, was obviously designed for grade-school campers rather than middle-aged cripples—and the quiet despair of mealtime, which began with each caretaker balancing two plates of food and ended in silence. Rob and I slunk out of the camp after one night.

Something shifted in me that weekend. I would be 50 in two weeks. Would I spend the next 30 years of my life suffering through silent mealtimes, cutting Rob's meat and trying to decipher a few tortured words between great chasms of quiet?

The reality had finally sunk in that this was my new husband: nonverbal, largely uncomprehending, exhausted, incapable of working, caring for kids, driving, or managing money. The girls were now 7 and 11—scared, clingy, acting out. Julia regularly threw tantrums and bugged her quieter sister; Grace had become a genius at verbally tormenting her younger sibling into a rage.

That fall I decided to go ahead with our long-planned kitchen remodeling project, the final design Rob had completed before his stroke. What seemed like an unnecessary complication to others felt like a vital step to me. Rob had hated our kitchen for so long. We had the money, so why not realize his final architectural plans for a room filled with pale maple cabinets and a glowing gold glass backsplash—the plans he had so lovingly crafted for our own home? We moved into a furnished apartment for two months, adding to our family's stress.

Suddenly I snapped out of my yearlong stupor. Since that hot July day when Rob tumbled to the floor, I had been putting one foot in front of the other, completing an endless list of tasks: get Rob into rehab, check; hire a nanny, check; apply for disability, check; find a job closer to home, check. Now that we had landed in what was apparently our new life, instead of feeling settled, I felt trapped.

A former neighbor, recently separated from his wife, had begun emailing me and inviting me to lunch. What started out as old friends commiserating turned into a flirtation—a flirtation that never went anywhere, though not by my choice. His therapist had warned him off me, a woman enmeshed in a complicated situation, and he had wisely listened. But just the whiff of possibility of a whole relationship with a man was intoxicating.

Over the next four months I acquired the name of a divorce lawyer who specialized in cases where one partner was disabled; toured a possible apartment for Rob down the street; and dragged him to couples counseling, even though he could barely speak. I also talked with a woman who had recently divorced her brain-damaged husband. When we met in a nearby coffee shop, she opened the conversation by saying: "I asked my son what I should tell you, and he said, 'Divorce is terrible for kids and everyone. Don't do it unless you have to.'" Important cautionary words from a family that had been there, but instead of taking it in, I was angry to be thwarted just when I had expected encouragement.

Undaunted, I broached the idea of divorce with Rob. I laid out my struggles with our relationship, my overwhelming loneliness, and my ideas for our splitting up. He sat there in silence, of course. At this point, he could barely string together four words, even under the best of circumstances. How could he mount his own verbal defense when I'd just flattened him? His face told me he was devastated by the very idea of divorce. How was he supposed to manage on his own, and what kind of lonely life would I be consigning him to?

But my thoughts at that time were mostly of myself. The girls certainly didn't want to live apart from their father. I was even desperate enough to approach Grace, then just 11, to ask for her reaction to a divorce. She, wiser than her mother, told me straight out: "I just can't deal with that right now, Mom."

As for Rob, Grace, Julia, and I were all he had. His mother and sister lived hours away and would be unable or unwilling to take him in, many of his friends had disappeared, his work had vanished. We were his whole life, and here I was, threatening to destroy that, too.

Two weeks later, on a snowy day in late January, one of our ministers called me at work. Pastor Eric said that Rob had called him, distraught and mentioning suicide. Pastor Eric drove Rob to the same Fairview Southdale Hospital emergency room where he'd been taken after his stroke; I was to meet them there.

When I arrived at the draped-off emergency room and faced Robert, faced what my divorce musings had done to him, I was shocked out of my fantasies. The road ahead didn't suddenly appear any easier, and I knew Rob wouldn't magically transform back into his old self. But seeing him in that hospital bed, so small, alone, and hopeless, made my escape plans disappear. Robert had already lost so much—his architectural career, many of his friendships, his ability to drive, speak, understand, ski, kayak, play with our girls. And now I was threatening him with the loss of his marriage and family.

To say that I was horrified is an understatement. Yes, American culture tells us that we should always be completely fulfilled by marriage, and if we aren't, we should divorce and try again. But that route is only fair when both partners are healthy, fully competent adults, or when one partner is so mentally altered he won't notice the change. Rob, though verbally limited, nevertheless knew exactly what I was suggesting and what it would cost him.

So right there, under the harsh emergency room lights, I held Rob's hand and apologized for suggesting divorce. And promised I would never speak of it again.

At that moment, I did not magically become a martyr. I still felt scared, trapped, and very sorry for myself. And I knew that I would be taking my imperfect self along in the years ahead. But I also saw that we three—me, Grace, and Julia—were all Rob had. We were his lifeboat. And as the sole functioning adult in our family, I could not leave him to drown alone.

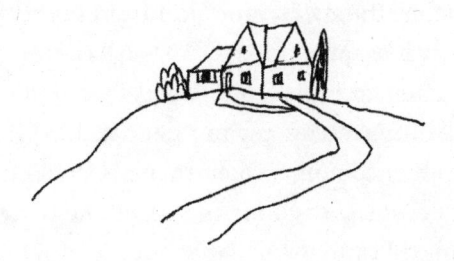

MOM'S DEATH

Although my mother had been diagnosed with stage four lung cancer in July 2006—a week before Rob's stroke—she managed fairly well until Christmas 2007. My older sister, Cynthia, spent that holiday with our parents, and it was then that she noticed a change for the worse in Mom.

I headed to Madison with Julia a week later and could see the shift myself since our last visit at Thanksgiving. Mom was far weaker and obviously in pain. Her doctor told us we should start hospice services, and as part of that process, suggested we visit Madison's serene new hospice building.

After getting Julia settled with a friend, the three of us toured the hospice. What a surreal experience to visit the place where you will die. We were polite, subdued, yet resolute in our mission, almost as if we were visiting a potential new apartment for Mom instead of the place where she would spend her final days.

We all nodded obediently as we were shown patient rooms, family lounges, kitchens, and other spaces, Mom taking the tour in a wheelchair. The windows were large and overlooked gardens and fields; the staff seemed kind and supportive. I knew that Rob's father had spent his last two weeks here, and his family had taken great comfort from it, but I wanted to scream in protest to be calmly viewing my mother's end-of-life site.

After we returned home, Mom turned uncharacteristically petulant. She complained to me that after she had written her college roommate Lyann to tell her about the cancer, all she had received in return was a catalog from Lyann's most recent art exhibit. I understood why Mom would be hurt, yet I was surprised to hear her complain about a friend. She rarely succumbed to the social pettiness most of us indulge in.

I knew it would be easy enough to track down Lyann at her New Jersey home. I called her later that day and told her that Mom was dying and would love to hear from her. She called shortly afterwards, and Mom was so happy to speak with her again.

I also contacted Mom's younger brother and sister and asked them to visit her in mid-February, around the time of her 76th birthday, which would also be the next time I was in town.

At the end of January, my sisters and I rendezvoused in Minneapolis to draw up a visitation schedule for the next few months. One of us would stay with Mom and Dad each weekend. We optimistically set up a schedule that would run through April.

When I returned to Madison in mid-February, Mom was clearly weaker, but her appetite remained good. She enjoyed the simple bacon and eggs or meatloaf meals I prepared, and was happy to visit with me as well as with her siblings and their spouses.

When we were alone, she showed me some bumps on her head—the cancer was now everywhere. I sympathized, of course, but never summoned the courage to ask her how she really felt. Was she scared? Was she angry? What were her feelings about death? Did she, a devout, lifelong Catholic, still take comfort from God's promise of life after death? My dad had confided in me that Mom was having an unexpected crisis of faith, but I was too cowardly to broach the subject with her.

Instead of having those talks, or even more importantly, telling her clearly and directly everything she had meant to me, what a wonderful mother she had been, and how much I loved her, I scurried around cleaning and cooking and making phone calls. "Mom, do you want soup tonight?" I'd ask as I whisked by her in the living room. "Is it time for your medicine? Shall we call your brother tonight?" I would do anything and everything except sit down next to her and acknowledge the inevitable.

When I left on that bleak February day, I confidently told my parents I would see them next in early March.

The following week we proceeded with a Mexican vacation—the first warm weather trip we'd had as a family since Rob's stroke. In some sort of haze of denial, I continued with the trip despite Mom's rapid decline. We returned to Minneapolis around the first of March.

The next weekend I was scheduled to visit my mom was March 7 through 10. On the night of Tuesday, March 4, a neurologist friend of my parents visited and told Dad it was time to take Mom to hospice. Because my father-in-law had spent a full two weeks at the same hospice, I assumed Mom would be there at least that long. Two nights later, on Thursday, March 6 at 6 p.m., Dad called to tell me that the staff was predicting Mom only had two or three more days to live.

Because I was booked on a flight the very next morning, I assumed I would easily make it there in time to tell my mother goodbye. I was wrong. At 7 that Friday morning, just as I was zipping up my suitcase, my father called to tell me that Mom had died early that morning, alone in her room.

I was overcome by guilt and grief. Why hadn't I rushed to Madison the instant I heard she was in hospice? Why hadn't I spent more time with her in the 20 months since her diagnosis?

Obviously, Rob's condition and the girls' needs were big reasons, but if I was truthful with myself, I knew that those weren't the only explanations. I was so overwhelmed by caretaking and so conflicted about my future that I simply did not have the emotional bandwidth to spend more time with my dying mother. And, like my sisters and father, I was in denial that she was actually dying and would soon be gone. It was far easier to maintain that denial if I stayed home.

Just a few hours later, I arrived at the funeral home to kiss my mother goodbye on her now icy cheek. Cynthia and her husband, Gary, arrived shortly afterwards. That night I slept alone in the room next to theirs and listened as my weeping older sister was comforted by her husband. Meanwhile, back in Minneapolis, my own husband could neither talk nor drive, so I had to ask our nanny Kelsey to buy dress clothes for the girls, pack everyone up, and drive them to Madison for the funeral.

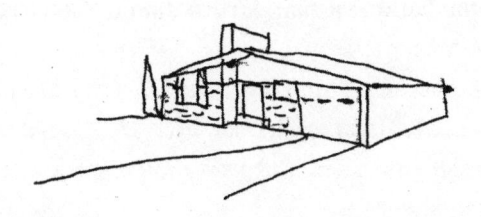

WRONG ANSWER

The following summer, two years after Rob's stroke, I decided to get honest in print about a few things. So, I wrote an essay for the *Minnesota Alumni* magazine (later republished in *MinnPost*) called "Wrong Answer." I've reprinted a portion of it here:

If you ask me how my husband Rob is doing—two years after his head blew up on our bathroom floor—I'd say, "Better," I'd say, "He talks more," I'd say, "a big improvement from how he was at first." I'd say that but I'd be thinking something else. I'd be thinking, "Pretty damn bad if you know what he used to be." Smart. Funny. Articulate. Busy.

But I don't say that because people's faces drop when I do, they get nervous, it wrecks the social equilibrium. I don't say that because my mother taught me not to say things that make people uncomfortable. Keep things light.

So, I go with the easy answer, the one they want to hear, the one that lets them still go to the movies or walk their dog without a cloud of fear wrecking their day. Because how can they keep drinking their soy mochas and power strolling the lake if they think their heads could suddenly explode, leaving them twitching in the fetal position by the bathroom tub? Struck dumb. Crippled. Locked up with geezers.

So, no. I don't say it all. I don't say: He talks like a drunk. Or: He can't talk at all. He wipes out on the ice. He hits the sack at 8. His architecture days are over. I don't say: You're a coward. Why don't you ask him yourself?

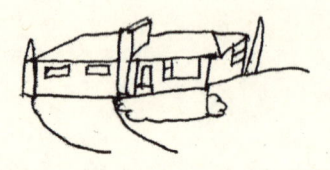

JULIA

And where were our girls in all this? Obviously, I was getting them to school, hiring warm and responsible afternoon nannies, helping them with homework, making [admittedly subpar] school lunches, even getting them to violin lessons and choirs and camps.

But between Rob's needs and my mother's death, I could see I wasn't focusing on Grace and Julia enough. Grace was often angry and taking it out on her younger sister; Julia was having tantrums and acting out. Both of them refused to talk with a therapist. Julia was not a verbal child, so her anger and pain came out physically. She crashed around rooms, threw things. One of our nannies, who happened to be studying occupational therapy, suggested a different kind of treatment called body-mind centering, in which the therapist takes the patient through physical movements to work out their psychological issues.

Julia went to a talented body-mind centering practitioner for several years, and though I still can't explain how it works, I know it does.

Nevertheless, by the time Julia reached the end of second grade—just 22 months after Rob's stroke—she was facing another problem: she couldn't read. Because both girls attended a Waldorf school, whose pedagogy doesn't emphasize early reading, we had been lulled along by her teacher's lack of concern.

But I could see this wasn't just a matter of being late to learn to read: Julia really couldn't decipher words. What was worse, she knew it, and had already begun internalizing the idea that she was stupid. In Sunday school and other outside settings, she could see that others kids her age were reading easily.

So, in defiance of the complacent Waldorf staff, I hauled her in for testing at a for-profit learning center. But when Rob and I returned two weeks later for the results, I was totally unprepared for what they told us, which was that our daughter had tested at a very low reading level. Julia had severe dyslexia.

At which point I sobbed out some incomprehensible combination of "My husband had a stroke, my mom just died, what are we going to do?"

Naturally, the director had the answer: Full-time summer reading coaching at his learning center and then two hours of daily afterschool coaching, to the tune of $20,000 a year. As much as we all adored the warm, artsy atmosphere of her Waldorf school and Julia would have loved to stay there, this extracurricular reading coaching—on top of a full school day—seemed like an expensive and exhausting way to proceed.

Fortunately, we lived near a well-respected private school for kids with learning disabilities. Each class held a maximum of eight children, the teachers were well trained, and the results they routinely produced with their students were impressive. So it was that Julia transferred to Groves Academy, where she would spend most of the next six years.

Within weeks of starting third grade at Groves, Julia was happier and relieved. It was obvious that these teachers really knew how to help her learn to read. Just as encouraging, her self-esteem began to improve as she made progress in the classroom. Soon she was sounding out letters and then words, writing sentences, and mastering special learning methods that made her feel capable. It was a wonder and a relief to witness her scholarly unfolding.

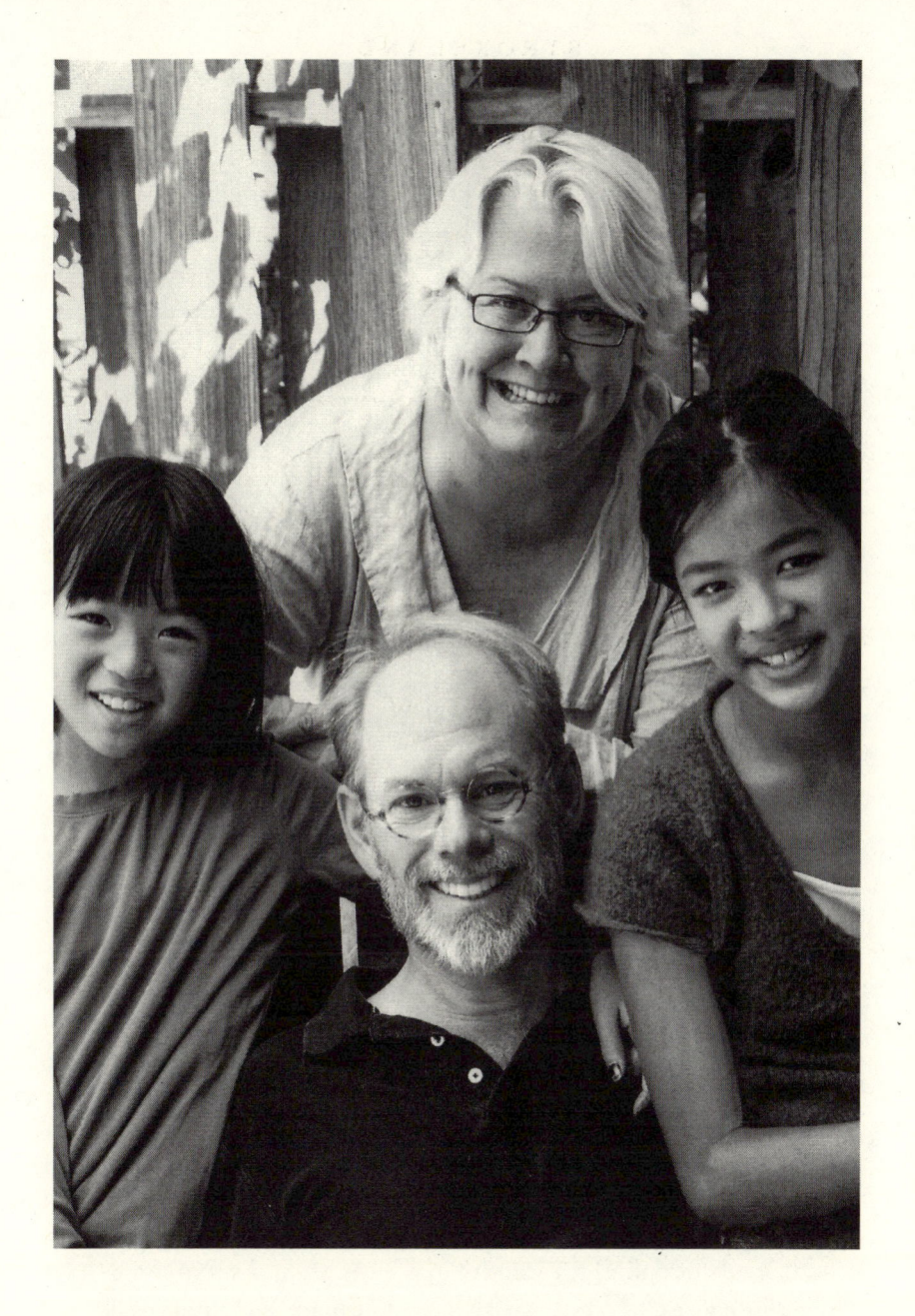

In the backyard of our longtime home in Summer 2008, two years after Rob's stroke (clockwise from top: Lynette, Grace, Rob, and Julia)
PHOTO BY CONNIE BICKMAN

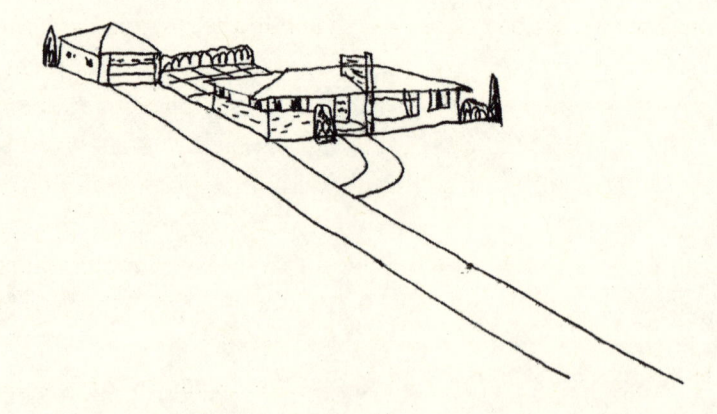

APHASIA, PART I

Rob stammers. He searches for words. The experts call it aphasia, defined by the National Aphasia Association as "an impairment of language, affecting the production or comprehension of speech and the ability to read or write." If you heard it, you might call it torture.

The pauses stretch and grow. At our house we know silence isn't golden, it's excruciating. Often incapable of waiting, too often I jump in, guessing wildly. I ask two, ten, twenty questions: What's the topic? The kids? The dog? The kitchen? The election? Is it good? Bad? Worrisome? All too frequently, Rob gives up. Never mind, he sighs. If the girls are there, they might remind me to give him time, to slow down.

For the first few years after his stroke, Rob suffered from both kinds of aphasia: receptive and expressive. Everyone notices the expressive kind, which means the person cannot speak (or write). But what was just as terrifying to Rob was the receptive kind: he didn't understand a single word that people were saying. And he couldn't read. Rob would often resort to drawing a picture of what he wanted to ask about: the car, the girls, the cats. Or together we would perform a strange form of charades. One of us would point to the fridge—is there some food in there that he wants? Then we'd lift out various cheeses and fruits until we got to the right one. Or if it was an emotion he wanted to convey, he might screw up his face and rub his eyes, as if he were crying. It wasn't fast, but between the pictures and the charades and Grace's almost mystical ability to decipher what her Dad was thinking, we usually got there eventually.

As the years went on, Rob began to understand what people were saying, as long as background noise was kept to a minimum, their speech wasn't too rapid, and the subject wasn't changed too quickly. Reading came more slowly, but was helped along by audio books, which he often listened to as he followed along on his Kindle.

But expressive speech—the ability to write and, more importantly, to speak—that has been hard won. In the rehab center, the speech therapists warned us that most left-brain stroke survivors, whose language center had been impaired, would at first produce only automatic speech, which resides in a different part of the brain. For many people, that includes shouting out "Hi!" or "Hello!" when someone walks in the room or a phone rings, and almost invariably, a lot of cursing.

Although I can't remember Rob writing anything in the earliest days following his stroke, my CaringBridge entries prove otherwise. On the sixth day following his stroke, I wrote: "Yesterday Rob indicated he wanted paper and pen, and using his left hand, wrote out a partial inquiry about work (I knew that would be his first worry!). We assured him all was taken care of, and then he wrote out a second inquiry about my job. It was so typical of Rob, the hardest worker in the family, to ask me why I was languishing around the hospital on a workday. And typical is quite comforting these days."

His writing at that point, of course, wasn't legible or fluid. In fact, Grace, our 10-year-old, had to decipher the word that he had intended to spell as Carleton, the college where I worked at the time. But he *was* communicating, however poorly, and looking back, I see that as a great triumph and a sign of the progress still to come.

Mostly, though, Rob got left out of the talking. It would be several years before he began deciphering spoken language and several more until he could follow most conversations. To this day, he poops out after about an hour of rapid-fire speaking among three or more people.

Aphasia is bad enough at home, but what about when Rob has to speak with a salesclerk, a teacher, or worse, an old friend? He watches as their eyes widen, mouths morphing into strained smiles—phony, pained. As their eyes dart toward the door, then back to me. Soon their questions are directed *only* to me. The conversation shifts completely, shuts out Rob as surely as if an invisible door had slammed shut.

He tries again to jump in, to interject. Their eyes flash back, panicked. Eyes he sees. Eyes that make him grow silent, and finally stop.

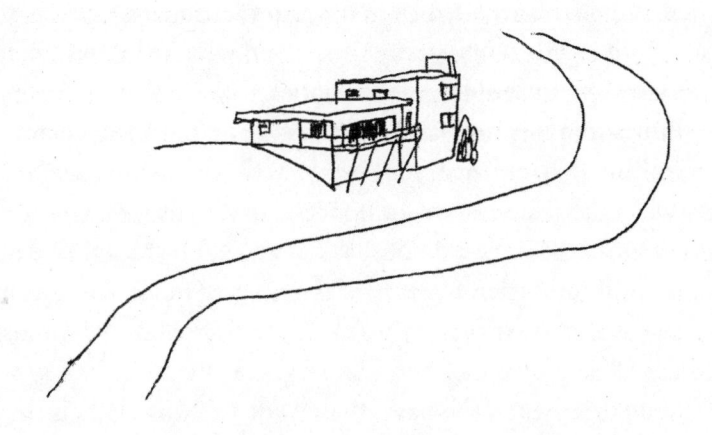

NOEL

There is a truism about friendship known to those of us whose family members have been very sick: Some of the people you least expect to show up will, and some of the people you most expect to see will disappear.

The outpouring of love and offers of support are greatest at the beginning of any crisis and tend to dwindle after a few months. That is unsurprising—human nature, really. When friends and acquaintances first learn of a medical issue, they rally round with lasagnas and daisies and hospital visits, with offers of childcare and yard help. But as the weeks and months go on, so too does life, and your family's health scare, however devastating, increasingly becomes the status quo.

What surprised me was not the work buddies and the neighbors who melted away, but the close friends who did. And of all those disappearing acts, by far the most painful was that of Rob's oldest friend, Noel. This was a man he'd known since high school, whom he'd visited often in various European cities, who had stayed in our home many times, and who had flown from Germany for our wedding. Poof. Gone.

But before he vanished, Noel made one last visit, about a month after Rob returned from rehab. At that point, Rob's expression was a glassy-eyed stare, he understood very little of what was said to him, and he could not speak at all. But he recognized all of his family and friends and he was overjoyed to see Noel again.

It was soon clear that joy wasn't mutual. Noel stayed for just one day. That afternoon, he and Robert did what they had so often done together in the past—they went walking. When they returned, I could see from Noel's frantic, darting eyes that he was freaked out by what the stroke had done to his old friend. Rob and I soon came to call this scared, get-me-out-of-here face the "deer in the headlights look."

Noel was sporting a serious case of dear-in-the-headlights, and my heart sank. I knew by that look, and by the speed with which he departed, that Noel would not stand beside Rob during his recovery. Noel was purely terrified, threatened by this evidence of life's fragility, unable to abide the reality of this neurological calamity. Noel was gone, and I feared he would remain so.

Sadly, I was right. Other than a few impersonal Christmas cards, Noel never contacted Robert again. Robert was sad, but I was furious. And on one particularly bad night about a year after Noel's last visit, I penned a scorched-earth missive detailing what a terrible person I thought he was, demanding to know how he could sleep at night after abandoning his old friend.

My sister Mary Beth, also a friend of Noel's, wrote him a similar letter, thus allowing Noel to blame the end of his relationship with Rob on the behavior of two crazy women. He told a mutual friend that we had poisoned their friendship.

I'm sure that explanation made Noel feel better about abandoning one of his closest friends, but the truth is this: neither Mary Beth nor I had ever spoken to Rob about Noel. We didn't have the heart to do so because we knew how much his disappearance had hurt Rob. When Noel's impersonal Christmas cards arrived, I watched as Rob glanced at them and tossed them into the trash.

Noel wasn't the only friend to dump Rob after his stroke—a regionally famous architect, once a close friend and colleague, also disappeared (this even after I wrote, imploring him to visit), as did many of the couples we'd once socialized with—but Noel's desertion was the most painful. This was a friendship that had survived decades and distance but couldn't survive disability.

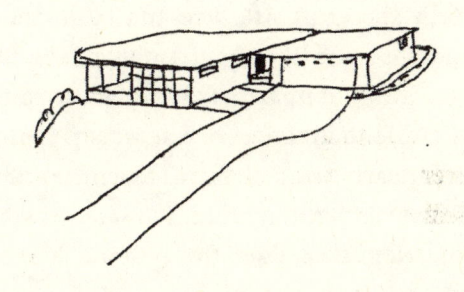

THE DAVIDS

While Rob was in architecture school, he shared a studio with three other guys, two of whom were named David. After college, the four of them stayed tight, and in the years since, they continued to meet regularly.

Dubbing themselves The Davids, they focused their meetings on touring a new Twin Cities building—a library, a museum—and then repairing to a coffee shop to critique the design. Sometimes they would discuss personal matters, such as family, but mostly they confined themselves to the good points, and especially the failings, of the buildings they had just toured. Architects are trained to be critical, and nothing was more fun for these guys than dissecting the design flaws of our city's latest edifice.

When Rob had his stroke and went through rehab, these meetings were suspended for many months. It must have been especially tough for his three college friends to see the toll the stroke had taken on Rob. Once the most idea-filled and articulate member of the group, he was all but mute those first months, struggling even to follow their conversation.

Oh, but how he looked forward to those meetings. The chance to talk about architecture and be in the company of longtime buddies acted like a tonic on Rob. He always returned from their meetings lit up by architecture and comradeship.

When COVID-19 hit in 2020, The Davids switched to Zoom calls. It wasn't nearly as much fun as touring buildings and criticizing them over coffee, but for me it offered a rare glimpse into their abiding friendship. Even through the door of his study, I could hear how Rob's laughter changed as he spoke with these men he'd loved for decades.

Their meetings did me good, too. The loyalty of The Davids has gone a long way toward softening my cynicism about the fate of friendship in the face of disability.

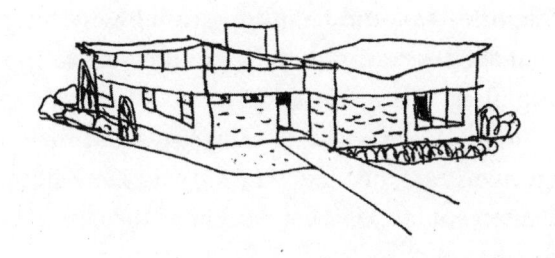

THERAPY

The therapist I went to for several years was one who specialized in grief. Although most of her patients had suffered a death in their immediate family, I figured my own grief was deep enough to qualify.

S was tall, slim, and fashionably dressed, with long legs she wound beneath herself on the chair as we talked in her light-filled office. She had lots of pillows for clients to clutch and many strategically positioned boxes of tissues. I went through plenty.

I saw S for several years, and it was helpful for two reasons: I could cry as much as I wanted, and she was a champion for me and me only.

I rarely broke down in front of family and friends, but the minute I sat down on her couch and S asked me an innocuous question such as, "How are you?" I would burst into tears and start snuffling and choking out things like, "It's har-ar-ar-d-d-"

or "I am so ti-i-i-r-r-ed." And then, weeping copiously, I would fill her in on the previous week's depressing events, such as watching Rob try to understand something the girls said or driving to Wisconsin to spend Thanksgiving with my dying mother.

One of the best things S did was allow me to admit to my worst impulses. Once she asked me, "When you're driving home from work, do you ever fantasize about how you could just keep on driving, heading west?" Wow. How did she know? Yes, as a matter of fact I *had* contemplated the notion of fleeing—many times.

Although I never left my family for good, I did take many trips in those first years, all of them encouraged by S. I know some of my friends, especially my stroke friends, were shocked by my forays to Arizona, Mexico, Guatemala, and India, but those escapes saved me and probably prevented me from becoming a complete self-pity machine.

On my first vacation escape, six months after Rob's stroke, I visited an old friend in Phoenix. It was January, deepest winter in Minnesota, but on her patio the air was warm and soft and so was the chaise lounge. Before long I had fallen asleep; I ended up napping for hours that first day, blessedly free from responsibilities and worries for the first time in months.

But as the years went on, and S could see I remained unhappy, she began championing a new cause—divorce. Our meetings became more predictable as our positions became more entrenched: she would argue that I could still take care of Rob after divorcing him, and I would argue that divorcing him would shatter him and blow up our daughters' world.

But it wasn't that impasse that ended our relationship. The end came when she launched a concerted campaign to improve my appearance. First, she recommended that I enroll in

Pilates, which she claimed had been a life changer for her. I dutifully attended a few sessions at a studio she recommended (in retrospect, a little boundary-less), but the machines designed to stretch and strengthen the body looked and felt more like torture devices to me. I found Pilates tedious and painful and couldn't wait for each session to end.

After I stopped attending Pilates, S revealed her true cause, which was not my fitness but my weight. I had gained 40 pounds since Rob's stroke. Because I didn't drink or smoke pot, food had become my drug of choice. I knew this wasn't great for my health, but given that my blood pressure, cholesterol, and blood sugar levels were all fine, losing weight didn't feel like my top priority.

But it was hers. One day, in a last-ditch effort to drill home how unsightly I had become, S said, "You could look so much younger than you do. You're only 54. All that weight you carry really ages you—it makes you look at least 10 years older than you are." Stunned and hurt, I could only mutter, "Yes, you're right. I really need to lose some weight. I know you're right...." My face flushed and my heartbeat quickened. Had my therapist, the person meant to support and encourage me, just told me that being fat was my biggest problem? I should have fought back against her sizeism and lack of empathy, but instead, embarrassed and confused, I let the hour sputter to a close.

But when I got home, I was furious. That session, that statement, and all the implied criticism that came before it was the very opposite of therapeutic—it was damaging. Our recent therapy had made me feel worse instead of better, and I was enraged by her "help."

So, I called S and left her a short message to that effect and fired her. She called me back several times, and even wrote me a long, apologetic letter, but I never spoke with her again. Years later, I am slightly embarrassed by my pique; it isn't like me to refuse to give someone a second chance. But S had betrayed our therapeutic relationship and kicked me when I was down. And that I just couldn't forgive.

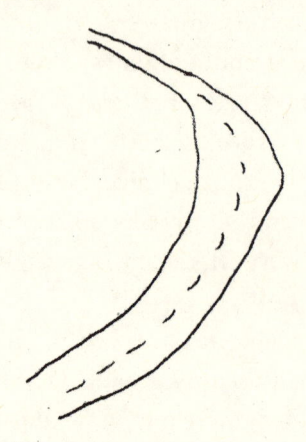

DRIVING

One of the toughest losses Rob faced was the ability to drive. This cut straight to the core of his independence. For the first few years following his stroke, he relied on me or on a network of friends to cart him to his many therapy appointments and speech groups.

From the start, he was determined to re-earn his license. I was worried, because his vision had been mildly affected by the stroke, and because I wasn't sure how good his reaction time would be in heavy traffic, or how he would manage to drive with the use of just one arm and one foot. He listened politely to my fretting, and then calmly went about the business of getting back behind the wheel.

Several years after his stroke, he studied for and retook the standardized written exam—no small feat for a man with aphasia. Here is the email he wrote me on the triumphant day in 2009 when he passed the written driving test:

> I WON! I WON! WHEW!
> YES. I WON THE DRIVEN.
> I WON THE CAR. I WON THE KEY.
> BUT:
> NOW TO BEGIN THE TRAINING.
> TO PUT OUT THE WHEEL AND THE THING FOR LEFT FEET.
> FIRST, GO BUY THEM. AND THEN BY THE 11/19/2009 TO TAKE IT AGAIN. SIGH....
> BUT, SAY EXCITING .... PLEASE!
> — ROBERT

And, just as he had predicted, we had our car fitted out with left-side controls, Rob took driving lessons at Courage Center, and he quickly passed his behind-the-wheel exam.

When he drove off for the first time, I'd never seen his smile so big. Freedom.

SUPPORT GROUPS

Sharing your misery is a peculiarly American occupation. The minute life makes you an unwilling member of some sad sack group—alkies, anorexics, Alzheimer's—everyone starts insisting that you join a support group.

Being the dutiful sort, I obeyed. Soon after Rob's stroke—two weeks? two months? Who can remember? — I trudged to a fluorescent-lit basement room in Fairview Southdale Hospital.

There, age 48, I sat with a tableful of blue-haired ladies. They were a decade or more past retirement while I—recklessly, stupidly, I now realized—was still parenting grade-schoolers.

At the end of the table sat the predictably earnest social worker with her inflexible agenda. Flashback to my husband pre-stroke: After months of adoption paperwork, Rob made me laugh by suggesting that perhaps to be licensed, social workers must first be proven humorless. The fiercely cheerful example that sat in front of us today was no exception. Between her jarringly upbeat tone and the room full of old women, I knew this support group held no support for me. I slunk out the door at the first break.

Through friends I met a few other middle-aged women whose husbands had also experienced bad strokes. Bad meaning left-brained. Bad meaning can't work, can't drive, can't talk. Soon five of us were meeting monthly at a dinner group I privately named the Stroke Wives Club.

At first it was helpful. Here, finally, were other women who got it, who understood what it was like to look into your husband's newly blank eyes, to try for patience when you're halfway out the door and your stuttering spouse starts to speak. It might take him 10 minutes to say we're out of milk.

But as the stroke wives kept meeting, I began to feel our differences. I was beating my fists against this new prison's walls. They seemed to be leaning into theirs. I hired nannies, gardeners, and cleaning ladies to give me time to breathe. They did it all themselves. I ran away for nights and weekends and fantasized about never coming back. They never left home without their husbands. I considered having an affair. They had pity sex. I dreamt of a partner who could travel and talk. They never admitted or said aloud what they must have thought at least once: *Please* let me shed this husk of a husband.

So many possibilities have slammed shut in our lives. I kept trying to pry open new ones. My fellow stroke wives couldn't or wouldn't, and their passivity and martyrdom began to frustrate me. Just because our husbands' worlds were constricted, must ours be as well? Would a *man* let his partner's medical disaster define his life?

I annoyed the other stroke wives by asking *why* they couldn't take that trip they longed for or attend that party without their husbands. I remember one dinner when P lamented that she could no longer visit friends' cabins because her husband couldn't hike, canoe, or swim. "But *you* still can!" I chirped. Later she mentioned that their son's home in Tokyo was too difficult a trip for her spouse. "So, go without him!" I cried. Her face dark, she answered back, "How would *you* feel if you were disabled and your spouse took off without you?" I said I hoped that, like Rob, I would be generous enough to encourage my partner to enjoy travel and sports while he still could. Wrong answer. By the end of dinner, my friends' faces told me they couldn't wait to get away from me.

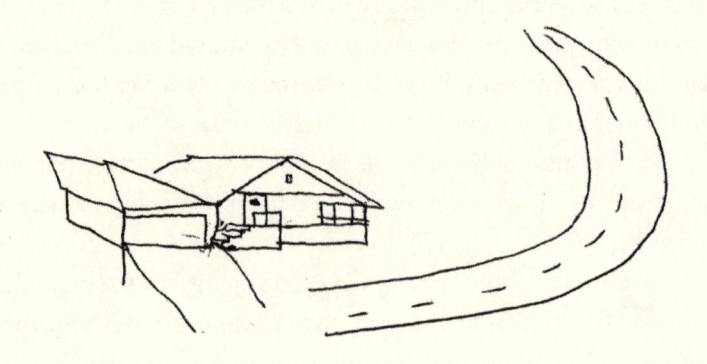

CHRONIC ILLNESS: WOMEN VERSUS MEN

I was surprised when I looked around the room of the stroke caregiver support group and realized that 80 percent of the members were women. Where were the men? Weren't women having strokes, too?

Yes, they are—even more of them, actually. According to the *Harvard Heart Letter*, each year 425,000 women have a stroke—55,000 more strokes than men have. But in the aphasia classes, the stroke support groups, even in the rehab centers, you see far more female care partners than male ones.

Why? Simple. Most men—especially younger men—are uninterested in being caretakers. They want a spouse who is firing on all cylinders. Thus, they are far more likely to divorce their chronically ill or disabled spouses than are women. In fact, a 2009 study published in the journal *Cancer* supplied these depressing statistics: A married woman diagnosed with a serious disease is six times more likely to be divorced or separated than a man with a similar diagnosis; among study participants, the divorce rate was 21 percent for seriously ill women and 3 percent for seriously ill men.

Among my coworkers was a man with young children who had divorced his brain-damaged wife, partly for financial reasons, and quickly remarried. No one thought any worse of him for it; indeed, he was encouraged to do so by all of his family and most of hers, and his new wife was welcomed into the fold.

I also thought of my two friends whose mothers had Alzheimer's disease, both of whose fathers started dating other women while their wives were still alive. When these fathers asked their adult children about it, most of the offspring had readily agreed to the arrangement. Would they have been equally understanding if it had been their mother who wanted to date while their father was alive?

A year after Rob's stroke, when I gently raised the question of divorce with a few friends and family members, I met with strong resistance. Even the colleague who had divorced his brain-damaged wife asked me why I was considering divorce so soon.

Men, especially those under 70, are not expected to devote their lives to sick or disabled wives. Instead, in our culture they are expected and even encouraged to move on. Few people question their need or right to do so.

The wife of a member of Rob's stroke class divorced him soon after his stroke, and if she is mentioned at all, it is with great scorn—both by other group members and their wives. My own sister was roundly criticized for divorcing her husband with dementia, even though his condition led to much chaos and discord.

Women are expected to transform, even sacrifice, their lives for a chronically ill or disabled spouse. Men are not, which explains why they are so rarely found in caretaking groups. My colleague with the brain-damaged wife was told by nearly everyone that he deserved love, companionship, and intimacy—a full life. Only my therapist ever said that to me.

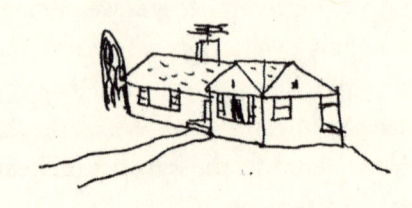

AMBIGUOUS LOSS

"Be patient toward all that is unsolved in your heart and try to love the questions themselves, like locked rooms and like books that are written in a very foreign tongue.... And the point is, to live everything. Live the questions now. Perhaps you will then gradually, without noticing it, live along some distant day into the answer."
—Rainer Maria Rilke

Before Rob's stroke, I was unfamiliar with the concept of ambiguous loss. Afterwards, I dwelt in it. Ambiguous loss, as defined by Pauline Boss, who described it in her book of the same name, is incomplete or uncertain loss, a kind of frozen grief. She writes, "Of all the losses experienced in personal relationships, ambiguous loss is the most devastating because it remains unclear, indeterminate."

The ambiguous loss I was living with was a psychological absence, or what Boss calls "goodbye without leaving.... a loved one is present, but his mind is not." Learning about this concept made me feel less crazy. It was strangely comforting to learn that many people deal with ambiguous loss, and that the pain of it can exceed that of a concrete loss, such as death.

In some ways, a stroke is even more ambiguous than other chronic illnesses because its losses change over time. I would find myself becoming hopeful as Rob understood more of the conversation, then desolate when he couldn't respond. He was there, living with the girls and me, part of our family, but in a completely different way from how he had been before.

Instead of an active, highly verbal, engaged professional and parent, we were left—at least at first—with a mostly silent, disabled man, incapable of multitasking, handling finances, keeping track of schedules, or doing much else beyond cleaning and dressing himself and preparing simple snacks.

I found myself yoked to a person utterly unlike the man I had married. The marital vows "for better or worse" take on a whole new meaning when the person you face across the dinner table struggles to speak. The man I had fallen in love with over conversation could no longer take part in one. Most days I felt less like a wife than the parent of three children—two of whom would grow up and leave home and one who would not.

It's not that Rob was childlike in his behavior. After a year of easy tears and frustration, he regained his emotional maturity. But he was childlike in his dependency on me, and that felt very unlike a partnership. Was I really married? Did I *truly* have a husband?

As the years went by, the ambiguity of our loss became more familiar and thus easier to live with. Although it has never resolved, because Rob has never fully recovered, both of us have found hope in other ways—in mentoring new stroke victims and their families, in making more friends in the stroke community, in raising our daughters and helping them thrive.

We also got better at communicating. Today it is not unusual for us to share a laugh over our dog's antics or to discuss a daughter's college challenges. Rob can't always express himself as well as he'd like to, but usually I can understand what he's getting at. If I don't, we keep at it until I do.

The various volunteer efforts I've gotten involved with through the years have helped too, bringing new meaning to my life, especially my support of groups in India and Guatemala, and my travel to those countries. I helped start a sponsorship program for a girls' group in India, which in turn has led to many more of the girls completing school, an effort that continues to this day. While in India I have taken them on field trips, done art projects with them, danced with them, attended their birthday parties. I have assisted Guatemalan families through financial aid, house building, and publicizing an important charity working on their behalf.

I knew that some of my friends thought I was a little crazy to hire nannies so I could fly halfway around the world to volunteer. But for me, these causes were a vital part of fashioning a new life for myself—something concrete that I could help fix, even if only in a small way, something to bring a fresh challenge and new energy to my days.

The profound loss from Rob's stroke has remained ambiguous, though the pain has lessened with the years. But out of this loss came new lives, and mine has included some truly rich challenges.

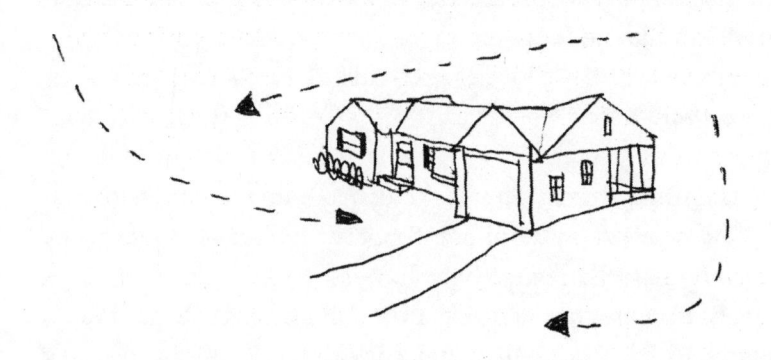

CARETAKING: THE MENTAL GAME

Articles about caretaking usually focus on the physical challenges of helping an aging or disabled family member: dressing, feeding, driving to doctors' appointments.

But in the 15 years since Robert suffered a stroke and I've been his caretaker it hasn't been the physical demands but the mental ones that have proven most onerous.

Like many mothers, of course, I have been the family's logistical expert, juggling in my head soccer practices, dentist appointments, school lunch fees. Then there's the to-do list that most couples share: arranging home repairs, preparing taxes, talking to teachers, paying bills, helping with homework. Single parents everywhere know the burden of doing it all, right?

So, it's not those tedious, everyday organizational challenges that made me crazy, endless though they sometimes felt. Instead, it's the whole range of extra incidents—mostly unpredictable but a regular part of living with a brain-damaged family member—that have brought stress and even terror into my otherwise mundane days.

To wit:

— The time, shortly after he returned home from rehab, that Rob threw away all of our Tupperware because some of the containers didn't match the lids.
— The time he chose a new dentist and proceeded to get $2,000 of [possibly optional] dental work done without mentioning it to me.
— The time his recumbent bicycle broke down on a remote path and he called me to rescue him but couldn't tell me where he was. And in my haste to find him, I managed to hit a kid on a bike (the kid was fine; I was not).
— The time he stopped taking his allergy medicine because it made him sleepy, and ended up wheezing and gasping in the ER, needing half a dozen more drugs and a dozen extra appointments to learn how to breathe again.
— The time he decided to stop taking his anti-seizure medicine (yes, it too made him tired) and suffered a full-fledged seizure while our 15-year-old was home alone with him. That incident ended in an ambulance ride and an overnight stay in the hospital.
— The time he threw away a year's worth of speech therapy receipts, just because. Taxes? What taxes?
— And the many, many times Rob has had something important to tell me—from the exact place in the house where the dog has peed to his desperate need for a new leg brace—but he couldn't come up with the right words to express it because of his aphasia. And I suck at guessing.

Staying one step ahead of Rob, reacting to various crises, and summoning the patience to wait out one more tortured storytelling—these are the truly exhausting parts of care-taking a brain-damaged spouse. Making dinner—that's the easy part.

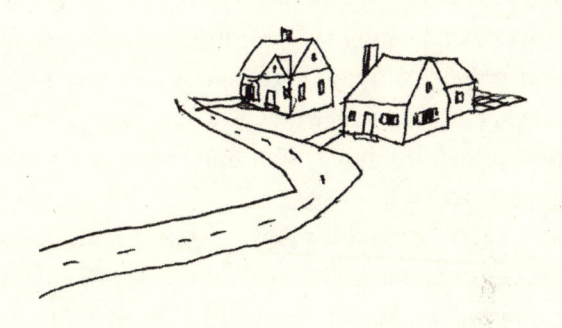

EXTRA PARENTS

One Mother's Day when the girls were still young, I received a call from a 21-year-old University of Minnesota student who wanted to wish me a happy Mother's Day.

The student was one of our nannies, Maddie, the latest in a string of resourceful young women I had found by placing classified ads in the *Minnesota Daily*. Each of our eight nannies was a hardworking University of Minnesota student who needed extra money. And each one of them saved my bacon.

Actually, our first nanny, Sara, was hired as a summertime convenience, as nannies are for many families—sort of a carefree alternative to day camp. Having her around the house simplified our lives, not unlike having a cleaning lady.

It was only a month after we hired our second nanny, Heidi, that Rob suffered his stroke. Overnight, childcare went from a convenience to a necessity. Our families lived out of state, so, unlike so many of my Twin Cities friends, I couldn't call on them to step in. Friends, of course, offered childcare and I took them up on the offers, but those playdates came one at a time and had to be constantly arranged. What I needed was regular, consistent help—help I paid for and could count on.

Heidi was that person that first summer, and I asked a lot of this 20-year-old girl/woman. Fortunately (for us if not for her), Heidi's family had experienced medical and mental health challenges during her childhood, so despite being young, she was strong and resilient.

In those early weeks after Rob's stroke, I asked her to drive our frightened kids to hospital visits, to lead park and mall outings, and to comfort them as their worlds turned upside down. I remember Julia, then 6, sitting on Heidi's lap and clinging to her, depending daily on her constancy and affection.

Later on, when things had settled down a bit, I still relied on our nannies for many parenting tasks— picking the girls up from school, helping with their homework, taking them to the dentist, even attending an occasional school event. Heidi, Maddie, Stephanie, Kelsey, Katie, Rachel, and Ashlee arranged playdates, oversaw school-supply shopping, refereed sibling squabbles, dried tears. My motto became, "I get by with a little help from my nannies." But in truth, most days it was more than a little.

When I was facing our first family vacation without Rob's help, Stephanie came along so I could relax. When Julia was afraid of the water, Heidi—a lifeguard who'd grown up on a lake—taught her how to swim.

I was glad to have help when 13-year-old Grace began experimenting with makeup and asking for friendship advice. Thank God for Ashlee, who was there to guide her through the thickets of female adolescence. After all, Ashlee had been through the whole ordeal herself just a few years earlier, whereas I had wielded my first tube of lipstick during the Nixon administration. And Katie was there to help two years later, when Grace had even more serious teenage concerns and wasn't comfortable coming to me with them.

Because Grace and Julia are adopted from China, I thought they could benefit from knowing an older Asian adoptee. Kelsey, a Korean adoptee, answered my carefully worded *Minnesota Daily* ad.

I guess it made sense, then, that I received that Mother's Day call. In a household like ours, so often fraught and overwhelmed, our nannies were more like extra parents or older sisters than household help.

Today, Grace is in graduate school studying cultural anthropology and planning to write her thesis on the racial identity of Asian American adoptees. Julia is a college junior majoring in chemistry and studio art. Both have far more compassion, insight, and thoughtfulness than do most people their age. It wasn't easy for them to grow up with a father who couldn't take them camping or talk with them about their problems at school. But they are fiercely protective of him and very aware of discrimination against and discounting of the disabled.

I am proud of the fine people our daughters have become, and so grateful for the young women who helped get them there.

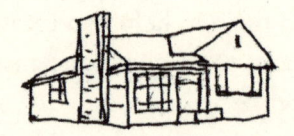

WHEN THE CARETAKER NEEDS CARE

It was a last-minute notion of mine that my high school freshman daughter Julia and I should take a small-group tour of Northern Ireland in April 2015. The teachers at her alternative school didn't seem to mind random absences, so off we went. But on the first day of the tour, thanks to one clumsy misstep getting out of a jeep, I found myself a patient at Belfast's Royal Victoria Hospital, a large metal halo attached to my triple-fractured ankle.

I was going to be here awhile, the doctors told me, since it would take another week for ice and elevation to bring down the swelling enough for them to perform the surgery I needed.

Meanwhile, Julia stayed with me while the rest of our group continued on with the tour. Julia, my exhausted, terrified teenager, doing her valiant best to comfort me, trying to sleep on a half-inch thick rubber mat while the nurses trod on her whenever they entered the room.

Despite how grown-up she was behaving—taking careful notes when the doctors came in, buying me pudding and juice in the hospital store, calling family members back home—I knew we needed an adult to help. And it was not possible for her father to be that person. He was incapable of traveling that far on his own, never mind navigating the medical system, the insurance companies, and the Irish accents. It pained me to remember all the times before his stroke when Rob had swooped in to save me during some minor medical emergency. Those days were over.

Rob would not be coming, so my intrepid world-traveling sister Mary Beth soon arrived, took Julia to a hotel, and I could let out my breath. Mary Beth began working the phones, and soon I was receiving texts and emails from friends and family, as well as flowers, muffins, and fresh nightgowns from her assaults on the local shops. Most importantly, she promised to escort Julia home.

The day before Mary Beth and Julia departed, my longtime friend Mary Griffin arrived in Belfast to take over. I knew I was lucky to have family like Julia and Mary Beth, and a friend like Mary, but an insistent part of me still longed for a husband who could rush to my rescue. What would happen when we got older? What if I got sick first? Questions like these cycled endlessly through my head as, night after night, I tried to fall sleep in the Royal Victoria.

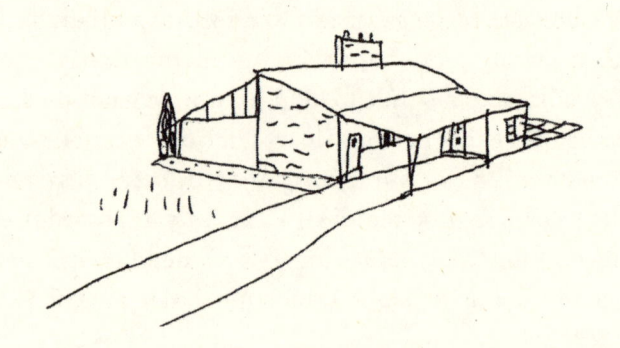

WHEN THE CARETAKER NEEDS CARE, ROUND 2

Four years later I needed to have that broken ankle replaced, and following surgery spend six weeks in a cast, boot, and crutches. Once again, I arranged for non-spousal care: from Grace, my older sister, Cynthia, and my college friend Diana.

The day before my boot was removed, we discovered that 75 percent of Rob's sinuses were blocked, and he would need sinus surgery the following week. When I wrote to my family about it, I included this postscript: "P.S. I get rid of my boot and crutches tomorrow, just in time to revert to caregiver."

Cynthia, who has always downplayed emotional matters, wrote back: "At least any caregiving you provide won't include a hospital stay or mobility issues on his part!"

Normally I would have let that comment pass but having spent the last half of my own recovery trying to manage Rob's sinus symptoms—which, like everything else in our lives was compounded by his aphasia, mental confusion, and impulsivity—I just couldn't let it go. I fired off a note to Cynthia that ended like this:

"Because on the surface, Rob seems to manage his daily life fairly well, most observers conclude that any caretaking on my part is no longer required. That couldn't be further from the truth.

"At the risk of sounding as if I am swamped in self-pity, I really want my sister, at least, to understand that."

My reaction, I think, goes to my frustration over how invisible caretaking becomes over the long haul. No, I don't have to change Rob's catheter, dress him, drive him to the store, or push his wheelchair. And for that I am grateful.

But the mental caregiving I described to Cynthia is unrelenting. No one else can communicate with Rob's doctors and therapists, file the taxes, pay the rent, figure out his medications, organize our vacations. Not to mention the daily game of "guess that question." What the hell is he trying to ask me, and how long will it take me to figure it out? Is it important or not? And how does it make Rob feel when I give up—or he does?

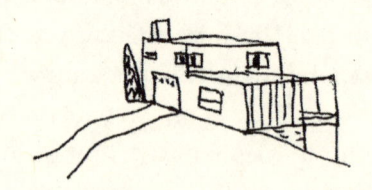

HAPPY ENDINGS, PART I

Two years after Rob's stroke, a book came out that made it impossible for him to be average.

In 2008, Dr. Jill Bolte Taylor, a neuroanatomist, published *My Stroke of Insight* about her triumph over the left-brain hemorrhagic stroke she suffered in her late thirties. Although Taylor didn't sugarcoat the devastation such a stroke can wreak, nor the profound fatigue and hard work that made up her recovery, her book's two major conclusions were not as helpful to her fellow stroke survivors as she may have assumed they would be.

Her first, and most memorable conclusion, was that—with plenty of hard work—even the victim of a left-brain stroke could return to their professional work. At the book's end, Taylor told of teaching university courses in anatomy and neurology, working as a consulting neuroanatomist, speaking around the country for the Harvard Brain Bank, and of course writing her book. Not to mention, cross-country skiing, waterskiing (!), jumping between rocks in Mexico, and a host of other activities most stroke survivors could only dream of.

She began chapter 15 by calling herself "grateful and amazed that I have *completely recovered* [italics mine] physically, cognitively, emotionally, and spiritually." Well, bully for her. And a great relief and comfort, I'm sure, to the thousands of healthy Americans who dread suffering a stroke and would prefer to assume that they, like Taylor, would emerge from it unscathed.

But for the millions of others, like Rob, who have worked just as hard as Taylor but never managed anything close to her recovery (and for their partners), the book was a slap in the face. Statistics show that only 10 percent of stroke victims recover completely, yet Taylor called that elusive possibility a likelihood, *if only people would rehabilitate thoroughly enough*, like her.

Her second conclusion was that strokes lead to a kind of spiritual nirvana. She posited that when the left brain—rational, methodical, analytical—suffers an insult, it allows the right side—creative, fluid, "connected to...deep inner peace"—to take over. Taylor described herself, even in those earliest frightening hours post-stroke, as feeling "both relief and joy," and her physical self as fluid, her "soul ... as big as the universe... frolicked with glee in a boundless sea."

Wow. Sounds like a really good drug trip. Unfortunately, that's a trip most stroke survivors I know never get to take. In her eighth year of recovery, now water-skiing and teaching about brains, Taylor wrote of longing for that post-stroke feeling of fluidity, sighing, "I miss the constant reminder that we are all one."

Must be nice. Rather than fluidity and one-ness, Rob's main post-stroke feelings were depression and frustration, his thoughts running more along the lines of, "Goddamn it. When will I be able to talk again?"

I'm sure it all happened to her, and every happy ending is encouraging. My problem with Taylor's book was that its immense popularity, coupled with its success-filled narrative, led to it becoming *the* defining stroke story of our times. Originally self-published, *My Stroke of Insight* was picked up by Viking, published in 30 countries, and became the top-selling stroke book on Amazon, its author a constant media presence for months. I cannot count the number of times her book has been recommended to me over the years.

Taylor's story—singular, rare, prized—became *the* story that every stroke survivor wanted to tell about themselves and the outcome that each of their friends wished for them—and now assumed they could attain.

And that was the problem: How many stroke survivors could or would have such an incredible outcome? Ten percent, at most, statistics tell us—and as our own experience confirmed.

I couldn't help comparing Taylor's campaign to the very different approach of a Lutheran pastor friend. Warren, like Taylor a thoroughly recovered stroke survivor, stopped making bedside visits to new stroke patients because he realized that his own happy outcome was unrealistic for most of them, and that holding himself up as a role model would only frustrate the very people he was trying to help.

Taylor's story confirmed the American mania for happy endings, as well as our nationally held delusion that anything can be achieved through hard work. Of course, often neither of these things is true. Because she insisted otherwise, while holding out false hope for stroke survivors, I grew to despise her book, which has remained the top-selling stroke memoir of all time.

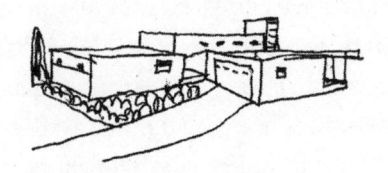

HAPPY ENDINGS, PART II

While driving in 2016 to a writing retreat with my teacher, Kate, and her friend Erin, a nurse practitioner, we began talking about our life stories as people do when they're getting to know each other. Erin asked what I was writing about, and I told her the story of Rob's stroke and his subsequent disability. I mentioned, as I sometimes do, that I wasn't home when the stroke happened, and that we didn't get him to the hospital for several hours.

Erin immediately launched into a story about shopping with a friend who started having atypical stroke symptoms. "I just knew she was having a stroke," Erin said, "and I rushed her right to the ER and insisted that they give her an MRI to check for a blood clot." The ER staff resisted at first, Erin went on, but, "a passing neurologist saw my friend walking sideways and agreed with me, they gave her an MRI, and I was right: she did have a blood clot."

Erin's story, of course, had a happy ending, with her friend promptly receiving a clot-dissolving drug, recovering completely, and returning to work within weeks.

And this story, like all happy-ending stroke tales, really pissed me off. Because of course I will never forget finding Rob curled up on our bathroom floor, never forget that I couldn't tell the doctors how long he'd been that way, never forget tearfully asking the neurologist if those few hours had made all the difference.

Haltingly, I tried to interject what that doctor—truthfully? Or just kindly?—had told me, which is that even stroke victims who are seen immediately don't always recover. But Erin brushed aside my interjection and repeated her friend's dramatic tale, in which she, of course, figured as heroine.

I could feel Kate's discomfort with the conversation, but she said nothing, clearly unsure how to intercede. I was a coward, too, as I so often am in these social situations. I listened once, twice, three times to Erin's dramatic retelling of a crisis averted, becoming angrier by the minute.

I know that most people prefer to hear stories like hers, stories with happy endings. I've known that ever since the first weeks after Rob's stroke, when friends kept cheerily inquiring, "How's Rob doing? When is he going back to work?" This when he was sitting in a wheelchair, mute.

And I know that most people, especially health care professionals like Erin, are desperate to think they are in control—that if only patients would get to the ER faster and see the right doctors, everything would turn out okay. Because it's scary to think that you or your husband or your child could be struck down at any time, and there's not a damn thing you could do about it.

So, I understood the impulse behind Erin's story, but I resented it all the same. What I wanted to say was, Please, shut up. Stop telling me this happy-ending stroke story. Think about how painful this must be for me to hear. I've just told you that I've spent years with a man who is a shell of his former self. Can't you understand from my weak responses that I can't listen to another minute of your triumphant tale?

I was angry at myself, as I so often am, for not saying what was on my mind. I spent most of the evening mentally composing responses to Erin, which I planned to level at her the next time I got her alone.

But in the end, I kept my peace. I didn't want to upset the harmony of the weekend, and I wasn't really sure it would sink in anyway. Erin was a golden retriever of a person, all motion and good spirits. I doubted she would really take in my reaction but would instead chalk it up to over-sensitivity.

I spent the rest of the weekend wary of Erin, despite her good nature. And I resolved that the very next time some well-meaning person told me a happy-ending stroke story, I would shatter the social niceties to tell them exactly what lies inside my breaking heart.

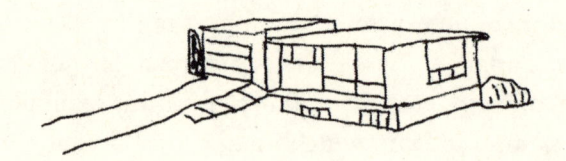

A CAREER CUT SHORT

A beautiful modern lake house designed for a sixty-something couple appeared in a 2019 article in the Minneapolis *Star Tribune*.

Robert spotted the story and marked it with a Post-it-note. He was excited to show me the article because many years earlier, he had designed a city home for the same couple. He was delighted to see their latest house and expected me to be equally excited.

Instead, I wept as I read the article.

An over-reaction? Probably. But sometimes, even more than a dozen years after Rob's stroke, the waste that is the loss of his profession can still stop me in my tracks.

Over a 20-year career he worked for a top residential firm, became a registered architect, opened his own successful practice, designed dozens of homes and remodeling projects, was named Minnesota Young Architect of the Year, spoke at conferences and on public radio, and produced plan books showing how to remodel classic American bungalows, ranches, and split levels.

He also designed a new kitchen for our 1902 Shingle-style house. That kitchen, a decade in the dreaming, would be Rob's final project. He finished the drawings three days before his stroke.

But our new kitchen wouldn't be the last reminder of Rob's professional losses.

Although we closed Robert Gerloff Residential Architects several months after Rob's stroke, five years later I was still fielding phone calls from potential clients. They had read about him in a design book, or in a saved newspaper clipping, or in a plan book from the library. Each of those phone calls was painful to receive, and then it hurt a little more when I heard myself tell them, no, Robert Gerloff wasn't working as an architect, and no, he never would again.

Then there were the well-meaning friends—I've lost count of how many—who quietly took me aside to ask if Rob could help them with "a small project" or "a couple of questions about our kitchen." I knew they were just trying to give Rob something of what he'd had before, but a tiny piece of me died each time I had to tell them no.

The reality of Rob's left-brain stroke is just as Dr. Seizert had predicted a few weeks after it happened: he has never again been able to communicate, design, or multitask well enough to work as an architect.

Today, at 60, he has renewed his subscription to *Metropolis* magazine, drives the long way home to check out buildings under construction, and avidly tours new libraries and museums with The Davids. Sometimes, in the privacy of his room, he even sketches little houses.

And like any architect, Rob continues to discover buildings he loves and those he hates, though it's much harder now for him to tell you why.

After my mini-breakdown over the former clients' lake house, I asked Rob if he, too, was sad about losing his profession. After a beat he said, "No. I'm just glad to be alive."

I am not quite so sanguine. Maybe because I remember more: his excitement when he plotted the hilltop site of my parents' new home; his passion to revive the humble bungalow; the look on his face when he first saw Palladio's Villa Rotunda. Maybe because I can still so easily conjure up the young architect with more ideas than there were hours in the day, confident that he, like so many in his profession, would keep right on working into his nineties.

Retirement, something Rob never aspired to, was forced on him at age 45. His profession came to a standstill on that hot July day. But his vocation? That abides.

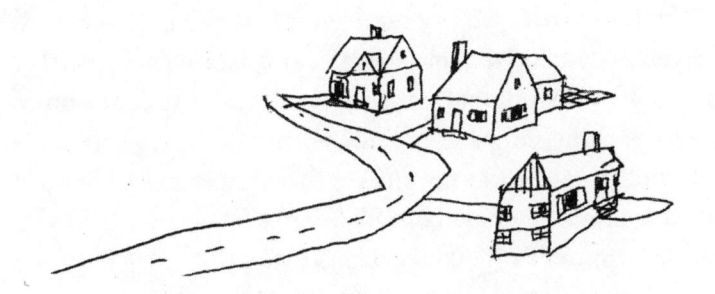

APHASIA TODAY

Even after 15 years, speaking is still tougher than writing for Rob, and sometimes the results are hilarious. He once famously began a story, "When I was a little girl…." But more often, the effect is intensely frustrating, both for him and anyone trying to understand him.

What is he trying to tell me? This problem is compounded by the fact that ever since his stroke (like many of his peers) he has confused the words *no* and *yes*. "Has the dog eaten yet?" "No, she has eaten," is very likely to be the response. So, which is it? Has she eaten or not? I sometimes want to scream.

Remembering and accessing proper names is still difficult for him too. It's one thing if he can't remember the first name of his new speech therapist; it's another thing entirely when he can't tell me the name of the medicine he just ran out of. When this happens, we usually resort to show and tell: He grabs the pill bottle in question, or we check the notes on his iPhone. Or failing that, he will literally draw me a picture. This is when his artistic skills really come in handy.

The stakes are especially high when we are discussing medical matters. Rob has terrible allergies and uses a whole panel of drugs to deal with them, ranging from pills to steroid sprays. When he is wheezing and gasping and I ask, "Have you taken the Ventolin yet?" he cannot answer that simple query but must instead lead me—by now both of us frustrated—into the bathroom so I can show him which drug I mean.

Even on his best days, Rob's tortured talking means he can rarely join in with group conversations. He also struggles to talk with just one other person, unless that person is patient and willing to slow down. Which rarely describes me. Our kids, now grown, frequently have to remind me to shut up, stop prompting his answers, and let him talk.

I mostly attend parties alone. Rob has given up on all but the tiniest gatherings—typically the two of us plus one other, well-known couple. Even at these small get-togethers, he can manage only about two hours before his eyes glaze over and the yawning begins. It's not that the conversation bores him, but rather that his brain is overtaxed by the rapid-fire talking that extroverts thrive on. It's a regular disappointment when—in the midst of an energetic discussion of local politics or work or kids—Rob pokes me under the table to tell me it's time to go home.

As many as 70 percent of all stroke survivors experience fatigue following a stroke, according to the Twin Cities newsletter *Stroke Connection*. Fatigue associated with the nervous system is hard for laypeople to understand, but it is chronic and very real.

And forget about noisy parties or restaurants—the resulting din acts as an assault on his brain. Rob cannot focus on one conversation when ten others are happening simultaneously nearby. Add in music or culinary chaos, and you have a recipe for brain overload.

That's one reason Rob avoids parties. The other is that almost no one bothers to talk with him. In any size group, most people find it awkward and uncomfortable to wait around while Rob attempts to articulate his thoughts. The process is just too slow and sad for all but the very kindest and most patient friends.

Aphasia creates a built-in conversational delay—sometimes brief, often lengthy—a significant pause between knowing what you want to say and figuring out how to say it. Parties, of course, don't work that way. People are focused on quick, charming small talk, updating each other about the office and the offspring, vacations and books. Rob's speech is never quick, and he has little to offer in the "what-I-achieved-lately" sweepstakes.

At a dinner party, I might interrupt the chit-chat if I can see that Rob is trying to interject a remark. I try to give him an opening, more time to say what he's struggling to communicate. But usually, unless we are dining with family members or close friends, he rarely attempts to speak. He can't bear the long-suffering looks pasted on people's faces when he tries to articulate an idea.

At large parties, I am as guilty as anyone of abandoning Rob in favor of chatting with others. An extrovert, I have always loved parties and am good at working a room. I am all too quick to leave Rob in a corner, even though it means he usually must remain there alone in strange, even threatening territory.

Nowadays, when I invite him to accompany me to a holiday gathering or large dinner party, he routinely says no thanks. I'm disappointed, even sad, but no longer surprised. I'm accustomed to attending parties alone.

Our friends should be used to this by now, too, yet I am regularly met with exclamations of dismay when I show up solo. "Why didn't Rob come along?" "We'd love to see him! Please tell him to come next time!" I try to explain about fatigue and brain overload, but what I want to say is: If he comes to your next party, will *you* talk with him? Will *you* give him the chance to tell you what's on his mind? Will *you* quash your own fears of disability long enough to seek out the intelligent, sensitive man who still lives inside him?

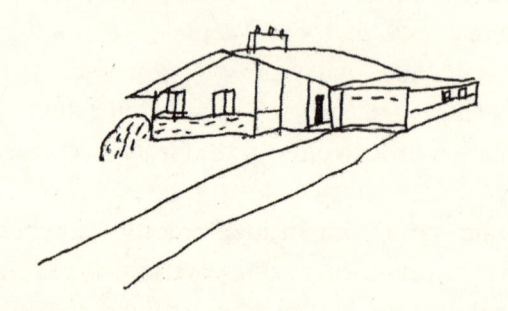

SMALL TRIUMPHS

In 2016, the Minnesota Literacy Council sponsored a night of readings to launch its publication of *Journeys*, a collection of writing by dozens of English as a Second Language learners.

In rooms scattered throughout the Minnesota History Center, immigrants from Nicaragua, Somalia, Vietnam, and many other nations read their poems and stories about fleeing war, living in refugee camps, and struggling to reach the United States.

Then there were the lifelong Americans, like Rob, whose native language was torn from them not by displacement but by brain injury. They read their moving stories haltingly but determinedly, or—as in Rob's case—stood by as another person read their piece. Here is an excerpt:

> WE BOUGHT A DOG NAMED ROSIE. ROSIE WAS SILENT, AND I WAS SILENT. I REALIZED WE BOTH GOT ALONG WELL BEING SILENT. I GOT UP IN THE MORNING AND ROSIE SAT NEXT TO HER BOWL, WAITING. ROSIE STOOD AT THE DOOR AND I OPENED UP. ROSIE LIVES WITH ME AND SITS ON MY LAP WHILE I READ A NOVEL AND PET ROSIE, CONTENTLY.

Small triumphs like this one are the new normal in Rob's life. What else makes up his days? Speech lessons with a rotating cast of university students, not all of them helpful, but Rob keeps signing up for lessons because he knows they learn from him. Regular coffee meetings with garrulous older people and other disabled folks in our apartment building. Weekly gatherings with two groups of fellow stroke survivors, who, like Rob, understand what it feels like to be left behind by the slipstream of humanity. These people have formed their own tight communities and lasting friendships—ones in which no one ever asks, "What do you *do*?" but asks instead, "How *are* you?"

What else? Laundry, dog walking, grocery shopping, errand running, reading, writing practice, listening to music.

And a kind of magical undivided attention, rare among parents today, that he beams onto Grace and Julia. When we gather, he is rapt, hanging onto their every word. He runs across the apartment every time Grace calls from Michigan. He is never too busy to drive Julia to a friend's house or pick up Grace's favorite chili noodles.

And that devotion, coupled with what his illness has required of them, has helped our daughters grow into thoughtful young adults. Ever since she was 6, Julia has been the one to wait for her dad when we're out walking, while the rest of us tend to forget and hurry ahead. On our first trip to Ireland when she was 13, Julia saved her dad's life more than once by grabbing his hand as he tried to cross the busy Dublin streets after looking the wrong way. As for Grace, she is fierce in defense of her father when we are confronted by impatient waiters or non-accessible buildings. They share an early maturity born of grief, loss, and the long struggle to relate to a disabled parent.

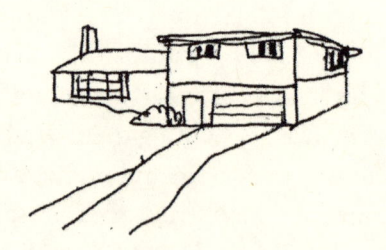

BIRTHDAY TANTRUM

A few years ago, after a few overlooked birthdays, I gave Rob and the girls my bottom line: A cake and a card. That's all I need, but please, do that much.

But in 2019, the first fall after both our daughters had left home, my birthday passed with barely a mention. By 8 p.m., I was feeling very sorry for myself indeed.

I stomped up to Rob and told him how ignored I felt—me, who like most mothers, was the founder of the feast for everyone else. Then I stormed back into the bedroom and slammed the door, feeing simultaneously ridiculous and justified.

Pretty soon I heard the apartment door close, and 20 minutes later, open again. Then Rob peeked into the bedroom to say, "I got you something." He had made a late-night trip to buy me a card and a purple orchid. Now I really felt silly. Had I just thrown a fit so my crippled husband felt duty-bound to shop for me at bedtime?

The next day I felt even worse when I received this note:

DEAR LYNETTE
I AM SORRY.
I AM BEYOND SORRY.
I KICK MYSELF.

I WANT TO BE INDEPENDENT—TALKING TO EVERYONE, MAKING DECISIONS, MAKING THEM LAUGH. I WANT TO BE INDEPENDENT, AND YET, I CAN'T TALK TO ANYONE, AND I HAVE TO COUNT ON YOU.

I WANT TO BE IN A RELATIONSHIP THAT IS 50/50.

THAT RELATIONSHIP,
OF THE WIFE AND HUSBAND,
IS SKEWED.

I WANT TO BE IN GIVING,
AT CHRISTMAS, ON BIRTHDAYS.
BUT I CAN'T THINK
TO THE FUTURE.
— ROB

I apologized and told him not to worry about it. Birthdays shouldn't be a big deal by the time you're 60. I have thought a lot about that night and that note. I, too, wish to be in a 50/50 relationship. But we are not in one and never will be. Only one of us can think to the future.

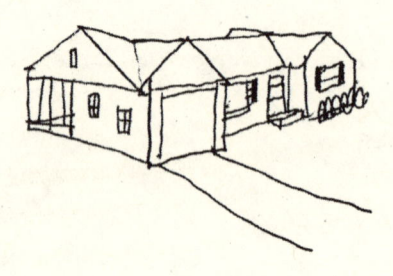

SPEECH CLASS

I don't often see Rob with his stroke friends, so it was a revelation to watch them together at a MnCAN (Minnesota Connect Aphasia Now) meeting in late 2019. In most group settings, Rob hangs back and keeps quiet. The rapid flow of conversation isn't easy for him with his halting speech, so after a few thwarted attempts, he clams up.

Not so at this MnCAN meeting, where he lit up the very instant we entered the room, animatedly greeting each person in turn. The day's ice breaker involved sharing old photos of yourself or your pets, and 69-year-old Bruce cracked up the room with a photo of himself at 19, clad only in boxer shorts, his hair styled in an impressive Afro.

In fact, laughter rang out repeatedly during the 90-minute meeting, as photos of dogs and 1970s teenagers circled the room. The formerly busy lives of these stroke survivors may have telescoped down into weekly meetings in a nursing-home basement, yet they seemed happy and even relieved to be there. They obviously shared a comfort level with each other that doesn't exist for them with civilians. I had rarely seen Rob look so relaxed.

Once the snacks arrived, the meeting dissolved briefly into chaos ("Where's the popcorn?" "Pass that picture!") before speech therapy leader Carly gently moved the distractible stroke folks back on track.

Next, Mary Lou, an 80-year-old woman, asked each member, "What's your favorite Thanksgiving tradition?" Listening to their answers, which unspooled in fits and starts, agonizing pauses between the words, was excruciating. But only to me, I reminded myself. The stroke folks were fine, prompting their own speech by drawing numbers in the air or tracing letters on the tabletop, looking to one another for clues, getting running starts by using similar words. From Julie, triumphantly: "Kelsey... daughter... me... pie... tradition." From Rob: "Our girls come home."

A younger woman named Stacy stood out because of her discouragement. "It's hard, dammit, dammit, dammit," she said. "I love to cook but it's hard." And a bit later: "I can't say it!"

But everyone else in the group remained positive, and took turns encouraging Stacy to stay upbeat as well. Carly told me later that Rob was a group leader—a person others looked up to and admired for his persistent efforts to improve his speech over more than a dozen years.

It was good for me to see him this way again—as a relaxed, popular leader—after seeing him as limited for so long.

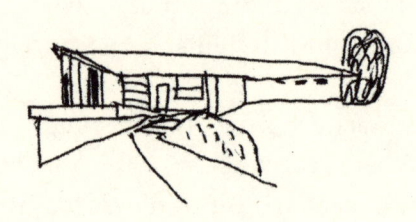

EMPTY NEST

When the girls left for college, the apartment got very quiet very fast. Suddenly the life I had signed up for years earlier became harder to bear. Dinner conversations were brief and disjointed, misunderstandings were frequent, vacations were lonely. And retirement, which had come on gradually and then all at once, loomed as a challenge instead of an opportunity.

How could I set up my life so that I consistently enjoyed the company of people other than Rob? What volunteer work would give my life shape and meaning now that I was rarely working as a journalist—a profession I had pursued for 45 years? How could we spend winter months in sunny climates without also spending endless days in silence?

More than a dozen years after Rob's stroke, I was accustomed to handling life's logistics—bills, taxes, moving preparations, health care—but I wasn't accustomed to the empty hours without conversation.

Suddenly I had a new understanding of the stroke partners who had left their marriages. In the end, it's not the extra work that will get to you. It's the extra quiet.

SENIOR STATESWOMAN OF STROKE

After I had been negotiating strokeland for a few years, I started receiving occasional phone calls from new caretakers, still reeling from the speed at which their lives had blown up and desperate for referrals, advice, answers.

The most recent such conference took place in 2020, when the 25-year-old daughter of a friend initiated a Zoom call from her home overseas. An aneurysm had burst in her mother's brain weeks earlier. A month later, her mom had left the hospital and persuaded the doctors she was fine. True, she was capable of walking and talking and reading, but she had more subtle, insidious damage to her frontal lobe. Everyone who knew her well could see that she was emotionally volatile and impulsive, except of course for the patient herself, who declared herself as good as new.

I was at a loss in advising this young woman. Rob had never denied the severity of his injury; indeed, he told me he knew from the first day that he would never work again. But this woman, a well-paid, busy human resources consultant, was certain that she would be diving right back into her frantic work world, despite the fact that she was screaming at people and bursting into tears a dozen times a day.

In the end, all I could recommend was that she receive an immediate neuropsychological examination so that she could understand the full extent of her brain damage; that she got plenty of rest (because all brain damage victims need that—Rob still naps daily); and that she avoid work for as long as possible. As for her young adult daughter, who was trying to manage both her mother's business and her medical issues from thousands of miles away, I reminded her that it was vital that she, too, get enough rest.

Finally, I advised her to contact the Minnesota Brain Injury Alliance, which educates and supports victims of strokes and other brain injuries, along with their family members.

But in throwing all this information at this young woman, who was barely out of college, I remembered how overwhelmed I'd felt in those first weeks after Rob's stroke. By day's end I would be exhausted from trying to field advice from well-meaning friends and attempting to at least note (if not actually follow up on) all the books and websites that people recommended. Most days it was all I could do to get the girls to school, visit Rob, and make a few phone calls about insurance. Becoming fully versed in the world of brain damage was beyond me, to say nothing of how damn depressing it was.

I'm not sure how much assistance I've given these people who have reached out to me. But even if I only provided an understanding ear and the chance to talk with someone who gets it, I hope I've helped a little.

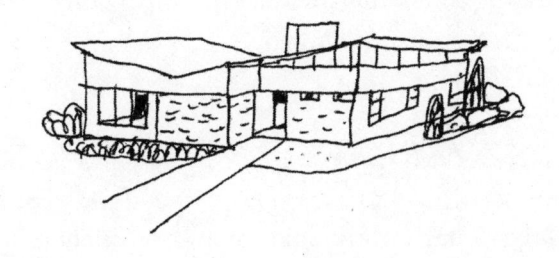

HALF A MARRIAGE

In the fall of 2020, I realized that I had been married to Stroke Rob for exactly as long as I had been married to Well Rob. I had spent 14 years with each version of my husband.

It's no wonder I can no longer remember what his voice sounded like, though I know it was low and soft, his conversation fluid and fascinating. Rob always had a good client story to tell, an interesting design to discuss, an insight into one of our daughters to share.

What remains? His warm laugh, his focused attention, his astute personal observations. The difference is that today, and for the last 14 years, Rob has not been able to convey those observations with anything approaching ease. He stammers, stops, searches for words, and too often, frustrated by the disconnect between his brain and his tongue, gives up.

Although we frequently sit together in the evenings in companionable silence, I can't deny how much I still miss Well Rob, and the talks we once shared. Ours was a conversation that I thought would last a lifetime. Instead, with each passing day, the marriage between me and Well Rob recedes, and the one between me and Stroke Rob becomes the only reality I remember.

STROKEVERSARY

Every July 16 our family holds a strange celebration we call Strokeversary. Yes, we actually mark the anniversary of Rob's 2006 stroke with a small party. It may sound morbid, but it's not. Cards may be exchanged, gifts may be given, but always we gather for dinner or an outing. In July 2020, we enjoyed Lebanese food and a soft summer evening boat ride on the Mississippi. As we drifted down the river, we reminisced about that life-altering time. "Remember the rubber duck we put in Dad's hand during the stroke so his nails wouldn't cut his skin?" Grace said, and Julia added, "How many times did we ride our bikes around the block, waiting for Mom to get home?"

We tend toward black humor on these occasions, but the laughs are really a celebration of our mutual survival. Obviously, we don't rejoice in the devastation inflicted on Rob's brain. Instead, we honor how much progress he's made, and the happy fact that he still lives and loves among us.

When we reminisce about that terrible time and the hard years that followed, we sometimes joke about misunderstandings born of aphasia. More often we speak of how far we have traveled since that desperate summer day. We are marking not the illness, but our triumph over it; not the disability, but the brave and loving man who emerged.

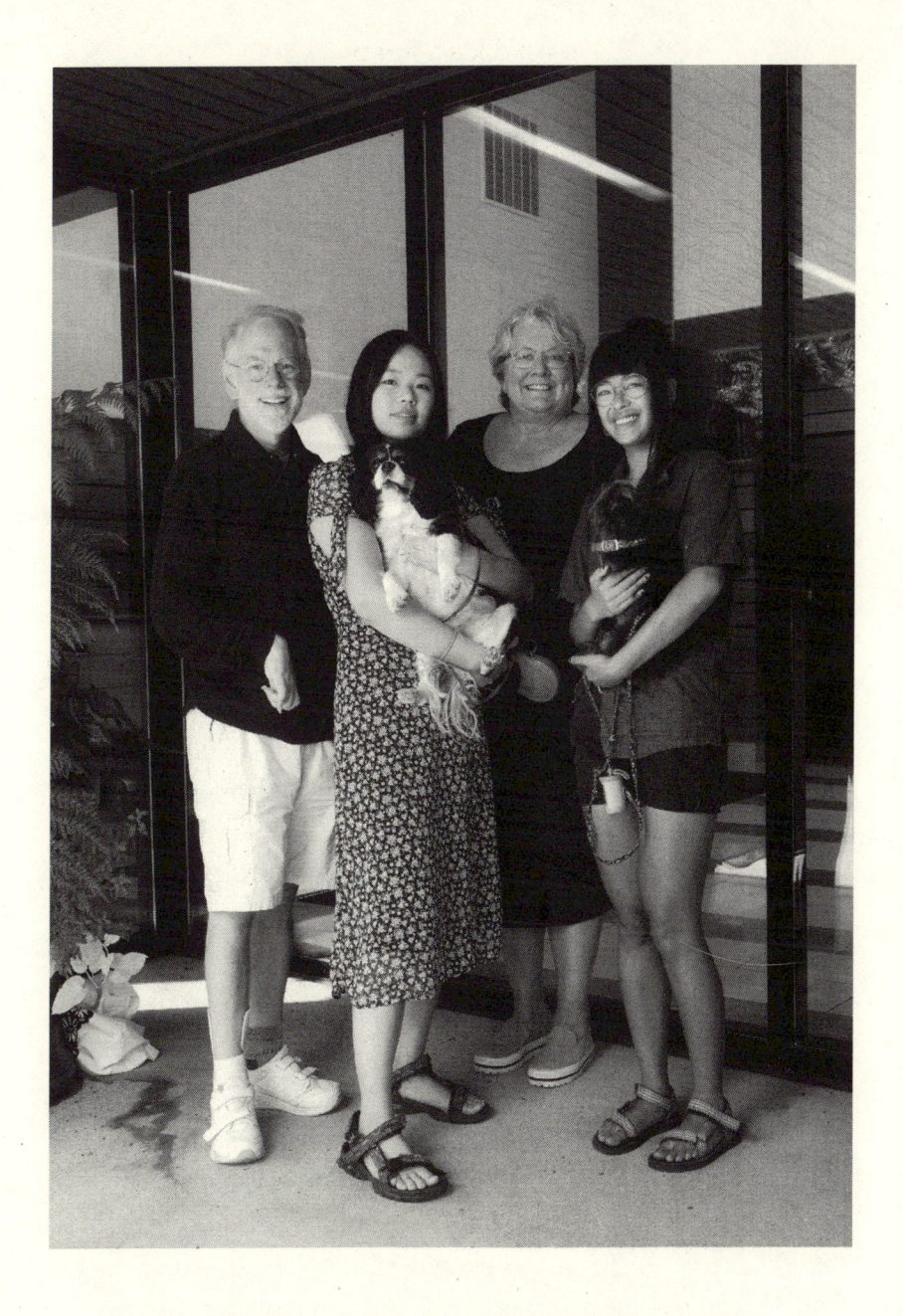

In front of our handicap accessible apartment building in Summer 2020 (from left: Rob, Julia holding Rosie, Lynette, Grace holding Angelika)
PHOTO BY SCOTT STREBLE

ACKNOWLEDGMENTS

Over Rob's long journey and mine, we have been lucky to receive so much love and support. Thanks go to:

- Our families, the Lambs and Gerloffs, especially Grace and Julia Gerloff
- Medical marvels, especially Dr. Bruce Idelkope, Dr. Barbara Seizert, and Carly Cauley
- Our ministers, Rev. Pam Fickenscher, Rev. Jen Nagel, and Rev. Eric Strand
- Our former nannies, especially Ashlee Siodlarz Balai, Heidi Flessert Columb, Stephanie Olson McRaith, and Madeline Simpson Schofield
- Our loyal friends, especially Faith Adams, Kristi Anderson, Karen Boyer, Diana Del Rosso, David and Grover Dimond, Mary Griffin, Eric Hanson, Julie and Jason Mascitti, David Malcolm Scott, Andy Steiner, and Jenny Werner
- Our girls' schools: City of Lakes Waldorf, Groves Academy, De LaSalle High School, and Perpich Center for Arts Education
- Our stroke friends, especially Janet Mills, Jeremy Holtzman, and Peg and Ed Pluimer
- And finally, the beloved teachers, editors, and friends who helped this book be born: Laurie Hertzel, Kate Hopper, Elizabeth Foy Larsen, Debra Monroe, and Jeannine Ouellette.

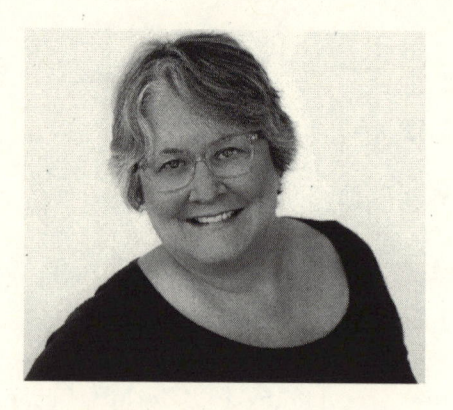

LYNETTE LAMB has been a magazine writer and editor for 35 years, including at *Utne Reader* and *Minnesota Monthly* magazines, and has been the spouse of a stroke survivor for 15 years. Lamb and her husband, ROBERT GERLOFF, are the parents of two adult daughters and live in Minneapolis.